Netter's
ATLAS *of* ANATOMY *for* SPEECH, SWALLOWING, *and* HEARING

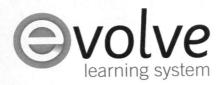

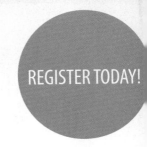
To access the free Evolve Resources, visit:

http://evolve.elsevier.com/McFarland/Netter

Evolve Student Resources for McFarland: *Netter's Atlas of Anatomy for Speech, Swallowing, and Hearing* offers the following features:

- **Self-Test Questions:** Approximately 150 practice questions with instant feedback, including rationales for correct answers, serve as an excellent study tool.

- **Labeling Exercises:** Key illustrations from the atlas form the basis of an interactive drag-and-drop exercise to help you master anatomy.

ELSEVIER

Netter's
ATLAS *of* ANATOMY *for* SPEECH, SWALLOWING, *and* HEARING

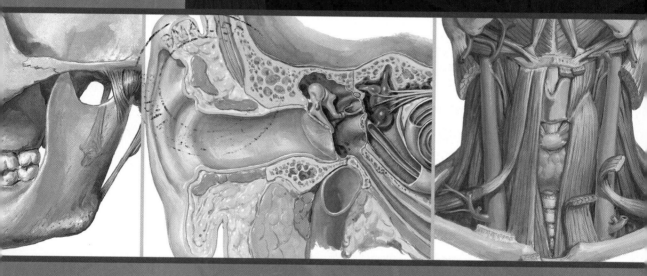

David H. McFarland, PhD
Professor
School of Speech-Language Pathology and Audiology
Faculty of Medicine
University of Montreal
Adjunct Professor
School of Communication Sciences and Disorders
Faculty of Medicine
McGill University
Montreal, Quebec, Canada

MOSBY
ELSEVIER

11830 Westline Industrial Drive
St. Louis, Missouri 63146

NETTER'S ATLAS OF ANATOMY FOR SPEECH,
SWALLOWING, AND HEARING

ISBN: 978-0-323-05656-4

L'anatomie en orthophonie: Parole, voix et déglutition © Elsevier Masson S.A.S., Paris 2006.

Library of Congress Cataloging-in-Publication Data

McFarland, David H.
   [L'anatomie en orthophonie. English.]
   Netter's atlas of anatomy for speech, swallowing, and hearing / David H. McFarland.
— 1st ed.
        p. ; cm.
   Includes index.
   Translation of: L'anatomie en orthophonie : parole, voix et déglutition.
Elsevier Masson S.A.S., Paris, 2006.
   ISBN 978-0-323-05656-4 (pbk. : alk. paper)   1.   Head—Anatomy—Atlases.
2.   Respiratory organs—Anatomy—Atlases. 3.   Speech—Atlases. 4.   Hearing—Atlases. 5.   Deglutition—
Atlases.   I. Netter, Frank H. (Frank Henry), 1906–1991.   II. McFarland, David H. Anatomie en orthophonie.
English   III. Title. IV. Title: Atlas of anatomy for speech, swallowing, and hearing.
   [DNLM: 1.   Respiratory System—anatomy & histology—Atlases. 2.   Respiratory
System—innervation—Atlases. 3.   Deglutition—Atlases. 4.   Ear—anatomy &
histology—Atlases. 5.   Ear—innervation—Atlases.   WF 17 M478L 2009a]
   QM251.M4413 2009
   611'.91—dc22

2008044248

Vice President and Publisher: Linda Duncan
Executive Editor: Kathy Falk
Managing Editor: Kristin Hebberd
Publishing Services Manager: Julie Eddy
Senior Project Manager: Laura Loveall
Designer: Margaret Reid

Printed in Canada

Last digit is the print number: 9 8 7 6 5 4 3 2 1

PREFACE

Speech, swallowing, and hearing are all human behaviors that are vital to everyday life. To diagnose and treat disordered function, you need a thorough understanding of the body systems involved in these complex coordinated behaviors. Such a background not only provides the basis of direct clinical intervention but also a common language of communication among medical and other professionals. The purpose of this atlas is to provide readers with a comprehensive reference for the essential aspects of speech, swallowing, and hearing anatomy. Key physiological and nervous system processes, which cannot be dissociated from their related anatomical structures, have also been summarized to deliver a more complete picture of these functions.

In designing this atlas, I carefully considered how I could best communicate such complex material to make it as real as possible for users. I had previously created a study text to accompany selected medical illustrations published by Frank Netter, which I provided as reference material in courses that I teach at the University of Montreal. Student reaction to these study tools was very positive, and this led to the idea that the format would be well suited for a larger work.

AUDIENCE

This atlas is for all those interested in the body systems involved in speech, swallowing, and hearing, either for understanding normal processes or as a basis for clinical practice. It is specifically tailored for instructors and students in both undergraduate and graduate education in speech, language, and hearing programs and also for researchers and clinicians in the fields of speech-language pathology, audiology, and related medical disciplines. My sincere ambition for this book is that it will serve as a useful learning tool for students and be a faithful reference for practitioners and researchers. I also hope that it will become a functional guide for clinicians who work with disorders of speech, swallowing, and hearing and can be used to educate patients suffering from these problems. Perhaps one day it may even become a platform for shared communication among the diverse professionals encountering the challenges of these complex disorders.

CONCEPT AND IMPORTANCE TO THE PROFESSION

This is the first time that the medical illustrations of Frank Netter have been gathered into a volume dedicated to speech, swallowing, and hearing. These seminal illustrations were chosen in part because they are used extensively in other disciplines and thereby represent a common base of study and clinical reference for students, instructors, and professionals in a variety of disciplines. The images also have garnered the favor of scholars and clinicians because they provide just the right level of detail and clearly convey the relationship among key anatomical structures.

ORGANIZATION

For the physiological component of the book, a similarly targeted approach was adopted to provide the essential information that would prove useful and appropriate for clinical practice. Clear parallels are made between the structure being referenced on the left page and the accompanying Netter illustration on the right. Each section concludes with summary tables featuring key muscles.

Ease of use was one of my primary organizational objectives. Because education is one of its primary purposes, the content is presented to match the way anatomy and physiology of speech are traditionally taught—from a basic introduction to anatomy to a more detailed discussion of the three key systems involved in speech, voice, and swallowing—namely the respiratory, phonatory, and articulatory systems. It concludes with the extremely important hearing and neurological systems.

DISTINCTIVE FEATURES

- *Full-Color Presentation:* This is the first and only full-color atlas of anatomy specific to speech, swallowing, and hearing, ensuring that the images convey the maximal detail and accuracy for students and clinicians studying these areas.
- *Stellar Art Program:* The remarkable, time-honored, and detailed images of renowned illustrator, Dr. Frank Netter, take center stage in this atlas. Dr. Netter's artwork has been used for years to teach leading healthcare professionals and researchers. Images presented from various orientations and levels of detail ensure that readers gain the foundation they need to work with patients who have disorders of speech, swallowing, and hearing.
- *Atlas Format:* The general setup of information presents targeted anatomical and related physiological information on the left page that corresponds to an image detailing the anatomy specific to this text on the right. This "read-it, see-it" approach appeals to a wide variety of learning styles and makes it ideal for clinical reference.
- *Instruction-Based Organization:* The organization of the sections within this atlas follows a logical order that is consistent with the way in which this content is taught in educational programs—beginning with an overview of anatomy and followed by successive sections detailing the anatomy and related physiology of the respiratory, phonatory, articulatory, auditory, and nervous systems—and makes it an ideal fit into any related course.
- *Appropriate Depth of Coverage:* The targeted sections of text—many presented in a bulleted-list style for easy reference and comprehension—present readers with the essential, need-to-know information relevant to speech, swallowing, and hearing mechanisms. This unique and focused approach provides just the right level of depth and detail to give the artwork proper context.
- *Summary Muscular Tables:* Each section concludes with the relevant musculature of that body system, detailing the origin, insertion, innervation, and action of each. These tables present vital information in a quick, easy, and consistent format ideal for study or quick reference.

ANCILLARIES

A companion Evolve website (http://evolve.elsevier.com/McFarland/Netter) has been developed to accompany this book with tools to enhance teaching for instructors and learning for students.

Instructor Resources

- *Image Collection:* All the images within the book are available online for download into PowerPoint or other presentation formats.
- *Test Bank:* Approximately 275 objective-style questions—multiple-choice, true/false, fill-in-the-blank, and matching—are provided, with accompanying rationales for correct answers and page-number or page-range references for remediation.
- *Animations:* Three-dimensional and narrated animations are available, focusing on the anatomy specific to speech, swallowing, and hearing and helping to bring the still images to life.
- *Dissection Videos:* Several clips from a live dissection video series are included, covering the head/neck, chest, and abdominal regions so that readers can clearly see the way in which the body's structures appear in context.

Student Resources

- *Self-Test Questions:* Approximately 150 objective-style questions—multiple-choice, true/false, fill-in-the-blank, and matching—are available for examination preparation and accompanied by instant feedback and remediation assistance.
- *Labeling Exercises:* Many of the book's illustrations are turned into interactive drag-and-drop exercises as a practice tool to help students ensure mastery of the relevant anatomy.

David H. McFarland

ACKNOWLEDGMENTS

This book is a direct result of my academic career—of teaching and research in speech, language, and swallowing. Many people provided support and encouragement during this fascinating journey—colleagues, friends, and family who are too numerous to mention by name.

I would, however, like to extend special thanks to Karyne Pelletier and Pascale Tremblay for their rigorous and untiring assistance, and to my academic and clinical colleagues, most notably Drs. Jody Kreiman, Christy Ludlow, Bonnie Martin-Harris, and Beth Strickland, who provided important critical readings of selected text.

My heartfelt thanks goes to Céline Armstrong for her long-standing support, and Kathy Falk, Kristin Hebberd, and Laura Loveall of Elsevier (USA) for their invaluable editorial assistance.

Finally, thanks to my students—past, present, and future—for the honor and privilege of teaching.

David H. McFarland

CONTENTS

INTRODUCTION

Speech differs from many other skilled human movements in that the goal is not to move the body or interact with an object but to communicate. It has been estimated that we may produce up to 15 speech sounds per second, which may require the activity of approximately 100 muscles distributed across the different physiological systems involved in speech production, including the respiratory, laryngeal, and oral-articulatory systems. The use of these different systems makes speech production one of the most complex of all human skilled movements. The underlying neural control processes are similarly complex and involve several hierarchically organized cortical and subcortical structures interacting with sensory feedback from peripheral speech structures. Swallowing uses many of these same complex anatomical and neural control processes involved in speech production.

The goal of this book is to summarize our current understanding of the anatomical basis of normal speech and swallowing function and to provide a platform for the diagnosis and treatment of disorders of these vital behaviors. Physiology is briefly summarized because structure and function are intimately related and are only artificially separated in this book to simplify learning.

This book is organized around the pioneering medical illustrations of Frank M. Netter, MD. Anatomical descriptions are presented with specific reference to these classic illustrations, and the relevant structures are highlighted. Understanding anatomy requires a visual representation of structure from various orientations, and Netter's figures provide this thorough perspective. Summary tables of muscle origin, insertion, innervation and function are provided throughout.

We begin with an overview of anatomical classifications systems, nomenclature, terms of direction and movement, and different anatomical tissues. We continue with descriptions of the respiratory, laryngeal, and oral-articulatory structures and end with hearing anatomy and key neurological systems involved in the control and coordination of speech and swallowing movements.

The study of anatomy is one of the oldest medical sciences, and its origins can be traced back to at least the early Greeks. You are embarking on this grand and noble tradition in the study of human anatomical principles.

■ ANATOMY

There are many ways of classifying and consequently studying anatomy. Some of these are described in the next sections. This book uses many of these methods to cover the following aspects of anatomy in relation to speech, swallowing, and hearing:
- The normal structure of organs and systems
- The topographical or anatomical relationships between structures
- The function of anatomical structures
- The development of anatomical structures and systems
- The neurological aspects of a structure's normal function
- Certain clinical aspects of disordered function

Systemic Anatomy

Systemic anatomy classifies the body by biological systems and sub-systems. The major systems include the integumentary system, the musculoskeletal system, the nervous system, the circulatory system, the respiratory system, the digestive system, the urinary system, and the reproductive system.

Regional Anatomy

Regional anatomy emphasizes the different regions or divisions of the body and the relationship between the anatomical structures of those divisions. The typical regions are as follows:
- Head and neck
- Back and extremities
- Thorax
- Abdomen
- Pelvis

Developmental Anatomy

Developmental anatomy concerns the prenatal and postnatal development of anatomical structures.

Functional Anatomy

Functional anatomy classifies the relationship between a structure and its function, combining anatomy and physiology.

Clinical Anatomy

Clinical anatomy emphasizes the relationship between anatomy and medical or other clinical practice.

■ NOMENCLATURE

Before beginning to discuss the human body, it is important to know the terms most frequently used by anatomists to describe a structure and its location. These terms greatly facilitate the understanding and study of anatomy.

Anatomical Position (see Figure 1, p. 5)

All structures are described in relationship to a standard position, which is called the *anatomical position*. In *humans,** the anatomical position is standing, facing the observer, arms along the body, palms turned forward, legs together or slightly separated, and feet straight ahead.

---

*Because most non-human animals are on all fours, their anatomical position and terms of direction are different from those for humans. This should be kept in mind when comparing non-human to human anatomy.

■ PLANES AND SECTIONS (Figure 1)

The body is described relative to different planes of orientation, and these can give rise to different sections or imaginary points of dissection. The three standard anatomical reference planes are as follows:

Sagittal

The sagittal plane is a longitudinal plane or section that is parallel to the sagittal suture of the skull. To visualize this plane, imagine a sheet of paper aligned vertically between your eyes. All sagittal sections are parallel to this sheet. The sagittal plane or section that divides the body into two equal left and right halves is called the *median* or *midsagittal* plane or section. All other sagittal planes or sections are termed *parasagittal,* or just *sagittal.*

Frontal or Coronal

The frontal, or coronal, plane is a longitudinal plane or section that crosses the sagittal plane at a right angle. To visualize this plane, imagine holding a piece of paper directly in front of you and parallel to the coronal or frontal suture of the cranium. All frontal sections will be parallel to this sheet. Coronal planes or sections divide the body front to back (anteriorly to posteriorly). The terms *midfrontal* or *midcoronal* are sometimes used to designate planes or sections that divide the body into equal anterior and posterior halves.

Transverse or Horizontal

The transverse, or horizontal, plane divides the body or structure into superior/inferior portions or sections. To visualize this plane, imagine a sheet of paper placed horizontally in front of your face that divides your head into upper and lower halves. All transverse sections are parallel to this sheet. The term *midtransverse* is used to designate the plane dividing the body into two equal superior and inferior halves.

NOTE: An oblique plane or section is oriented obliquely between one of the planes described here.

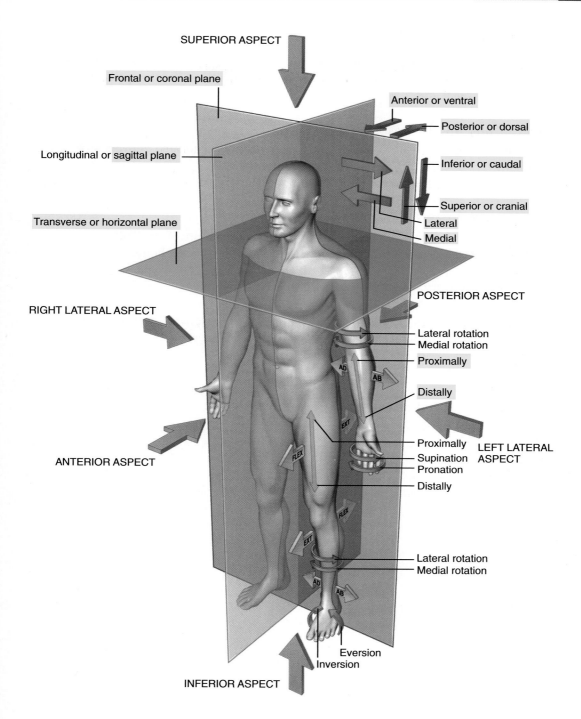

Figure 1. Anatomical position, terms of relationships, and body planes. (From Standring S: *Gray's anatomy: the anatomical basis of clinical practice,* ed 39, Edinburgh, 2005, Churchill Livingstone.)

■ ANATOMICAL TERMS

Directional terms are used to locate anatomical structures and to explain the spatial relationship between structures relative to the anatomical position. They are presented in contrasting pairs (see Figure 1, p. 5).

Superior and Inferior (Figure 2)

- Superior (rostral, cranial) is toward the upper portion or located above a structure of the body.
- Inferior (caudal) is toward the lower portion or below a structure of the body.

Anterior and Posterior (Figure 3, p. 8)

- Anterior (ventral) is toward the front or in front of a structure of the body.
- Posterior (dorsal) is toward the back or behind a structure of the body.

Medial, Lateral, and Median (Figure 4, p. 9)

- Medial is toward the midline, or central axis, of the body.
- Lateral is away from the central axis, or midline, of the body.
- Median is on the central sagittal plane.

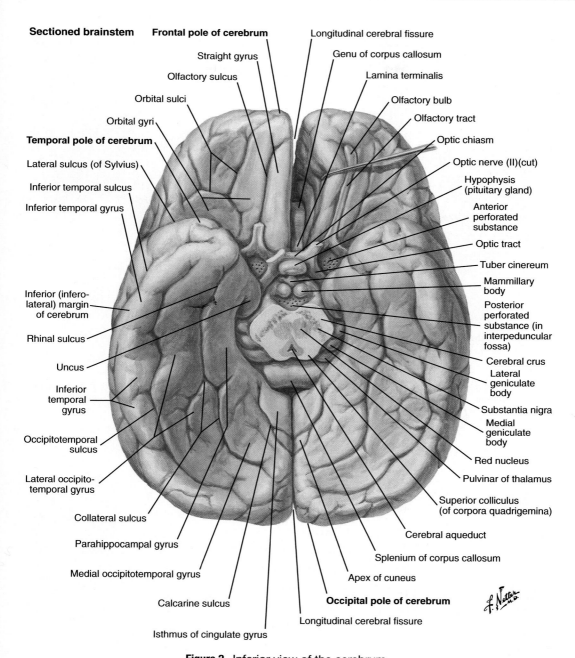

Sectioned brainstem

Frontal pole of cerebrum

Straight gyrus

Olfactory sulcus

Orbital sulci

Orbital gyri

Temporal pole of cerebrum

Lateral sulcus (of Sylvius)

Inferior temporal sulcus

Inferior temporal gyrus

Inferior (infero-
lateral) margin
of cerebrum

Rhinal sulcus

Uncus

Inferior
temporal
gyrus

Occipitotemporal
sulcus

Lateral occipito-
temporal gyrus

Collateral sulcus

Parahippocampal gyrus

Medial occipitotemporal gyrus

Calcarine sulcus

Isthmus of cingulate gyrus

Longitudinal cerebral fissure

Genu of corpus callosum

Lamina terminalis

Olfactory bulb

Olfactory tract

Optic chiasm

Optic nerve (II)(cut)

Hypophysis
(pituitary gland)

Anterior
perforated
substance

Optic tract

Tuber cinereum

Mammillary
body

Posterior
perforated
substance (in
interpeduncular
fossa)

Cerebral crus

Lateral
geniculate
body

Substantia nigra

Medial
geniculate
body

Red nucleus

Pulvinar of thalamus

Superior colliculus
(of corpora quadrigemina)

Cerebral aqueduct

Splenium of corpus callosum

Apex of cuneus

Occipital pole of cerebrum

Longitudinal cerebral fissure

Figure 2. Inferior view of the cerebrum.

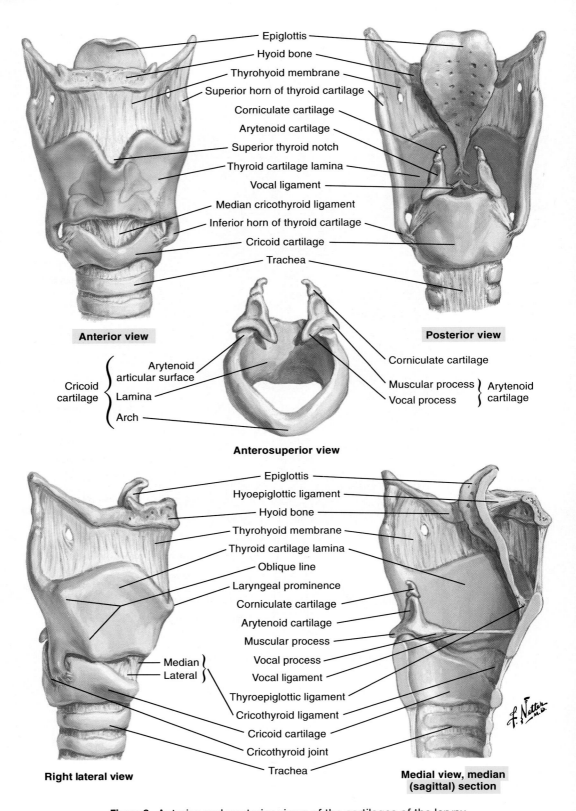

Anterior view

Epiglottis
Hyoid bone
Thyrohyoid membrane
Superior horn of thyroid cartilage
Corniculate cartilage
Arytenoid cartilage
Superior thyroid notch
Thyroid cartilage lamina
Vocal ligament
Median cricothyroid ligament
Inferior horn of thyroid cartilage
Cricoid cartilage
Trachea

Posterior view

Cricoid cartilage
- Arytenoid articular surface
- Lamina
- Arch

Corniculate cartilage
Muscular process
Vocal process
Arytenoid cartilage

Anterosuperior view

Epiglottis
Hyoepiglottic ligament
Hyoid bone
Thyrohyoid membrane
Thyroid cartilage lamina
Oblique line
Laryngeal prominence
Corniculate cartilage
Arytenoid cartilage
Muscular process
Vocal process
Vocal ligament
Thyroepiglottic ligament
Cricothyroid ligament
Cricoid cartilage
Cricothyroid joint
Trachea

Median
Lateral

Right lateral view

Medial view, median (sagittal) section

Figure 3. Anterior and posterior views of the cartilages of the larynx.

Legends of certain plates are highlighted in yellow to emphasize the related elements in the corresponding text.

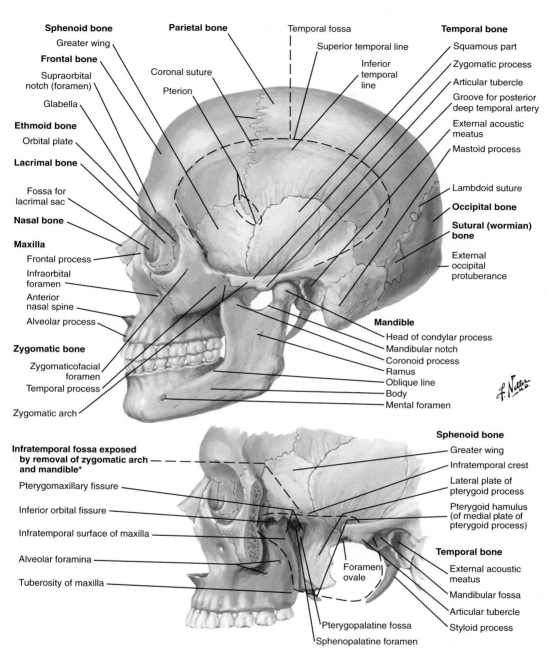

Sphenoid bone
Greater wing
Frontal bone
Supraorbital notch (foramen)
Glabella
Ethmoid bone
Orbital plate
Lacrimal bone
Fossa for lacrimal sac
Nasal bone
Maxilla
Frontal process
Infraorbital foramen
Anterior nasal spine
Alveolar process
Zygomatic bone
Zygomaticofacial foramen
Temporal process
Zygomatic arch

Parietal bone
Coronal suture
Pterion

Temporal fossa
Superior temporal line
Inferior temporal line

Temporal bone
Squamous part
Zygomatic process
Articular tubercle
Groove for posterior deep temporal artery
External acoustic meatus
Mastoid process
Lambdoid suture
Occipital bone
Sutural (wormian) bone
External occipital protuberance

Mandible
Head of condylar process
Mandibular notch
Coronoid process
Ramus
Oblique line
Body
Mental foramen

Infratemporal fossa exposed by removal of zygomatic arch and mandible*
Pterygomaxillary fissure
Inferior orbital fissure
Infratemporal surface of maxilla
Alveolar foramina
Tuberosity of maxilla

Foramen ovale

Pterygopalatine fossa
Sphenopalatine foramen

Sphenoid bone
Greater wing
Infratemporal crest
Lateral plate of pterygoid process
Pterygoid hamulus (of medial plate of pterygoid process)
Temporal bone
External acoustic meatus
Mandibular fossa
Articular tubercle
Styloid process

*Superficially, mastoid process forms posterior boundary.

Figure 4. Lateral view of the skull.

Proximal and Distal

- Proximal is toward the origin of a structure of the body.
- Distal is away from the origin of a structure of the body. Proximal and distal are often used to describe the limbs.

External, Internal, and Intermediate

- External (superficial) is toward the surface of a structure of the body.
- Internal (deep) is away from the surface of a structure of the body.
- Intermediate (middle) is in between internal and external.

These terms are often used to describe anatomical relationships between structures, such as one structure being deep to or superficial to another.

Parietal and Visceral (Figure 5)

- Parietal is the outer layer or covering of a body cavity.
- Visceral is the inner layer of a cavity wrapped around body organs.

Prone and Supine

- Prone is the anatomical position of the body with the face and ventral surface of the body facing down.
- Supine is the anatomical position of the body with the face and ventral surface of the body facing up.

Ipsilateral, Contralateral, and Bilateral

- Ipsilateral refers to the same side of the body.
- Contralateral refers to the opposite side of the body.
- Bilateral refers to both sides of the body.

■ VIEWS AND ASPECTS

Anatomy requires the visualization of structures from different perspectives. The terms view, aspect, and surface are used to describe these orientations. For example, an anterior view is when the observer is positioned anteriorly and looking posteriorly at a structure. An anterior aspect or surface of the structure would be in view (see Figures 1 [p. 5] and 5).

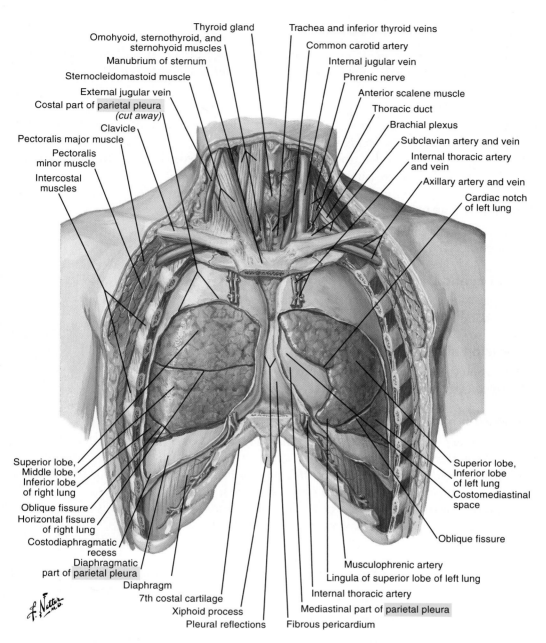

Thyroid gland
Omohyoid, sternothyroid, and sternohyoid muscles
Manubrium of sternum
Sternocleidomastoid muscle
External jugular vein
Costal part of parietal pleura (cut away)
Clavicle
Pectoralis major muscle
Pectoralis minor muscle
Intercostal muscles

Trachea and inferior thyroid veins
Common carotid artery
Internal jugular vein
Phrenic nerve
Anterior scalene muscle
Thoracic duct
Brachial plexus
Subclavian artery and vein
Internal thoracic artery and vein
Axillary artery and vein
Cardiac notch of left lung

Superior lobe,
Middle lobe,
Inferior lobe
of right lung
Oblique fissure
Horizontal fissure of right lung
Costodiaphragmatic recess
Diaphragmatic part of parietal pleura
Diaphragm
7th costal cartilage
Xiphoid process
Pleural reflections

Superior lobe,
Inferior lobe
of left lung
Costomediastinal space
Oblique fissure

Musculophrenic artery
Lingula of superior lobe of left lung
Internal thoracic artery
Mediastinal part of parietal pleura
Fibrous pericardium

Figure 5. Anterior view of the lungs in situ. Note the parietal pleura.

■ ANATOMICAL MOVEMENT

As with terms of direction, anatomical movements are usually described in contrasting pairs. Each pair is detailed in the following sections (see also Figure 1, p. 5).

Flexion and Extension

- Flexion is the movement around a joint that brings two adjacent bones or body segments closer together, reducing the angle of articulation.
- Extension is the movement around a joint that brings two adjacent bones or body segments farther apart, increasing the angle of articulation.

Abduction and Adduction

- Abduction is the movement of a structure away from the midline.
- Adduction is the movement of a structure toward the midline.

Elevation and Depression

- Elevation is the upward movement of a structure.
- Depression is the downward movement of a structure.

Protrusion and Retrusion

- Protrusion (protraction) is the forward movement of a structure.
- Retrusion (retraction) is the backward movement of a structure.

Supination and Pronation

Supination and pronation refer to rotational movements of certain structures such as the arm and hand:
- Supination refers to the rotation of the arm and hand so that the palm is facing anteriorly (with arm straight) or upward (with arm bent).
- Pronation refers to the rotation of the arm and hand so that the palm is facing posteriorly (with arm straight) or downward (with arm bent).

■ VOCABULARY SPECIFIC TO ANATOMY

Many structures are named according to either their anatomical location on the body (e.g., external intercostal muscles, supra glottic, and so on) or their function (e.g., levator scapulae muscle, depressor anguli oris muscle, and so on). In addition to their anatomical name, other structures have names originating from mythology (e.g., Achilles tendon) or from the first person who associated the structure to a disease or a malformation or the first person who described the structure (e.g., circle of Willis).

Names of muscles and ligaments correspond to their points of attachment, as follows:
- Origin corresponds to the point of attachment of a muscle that remains relatively fixed during muscular contraction.
- Insertion corresponds to the more mobile point of attachment.

In general, the origin is named first and the insertion second. Sometimes, origin and insertion can be interchanged (insertion first and origin second) if both are considered of equal mobility. Muscle names may also provide information about the form of the muscle such as the number of bellies or portions of the muscle (e.g., *di*gastric, or two bellies), its overall shape or location (e.g., external intercostals), or its action (e.g., *tensor* veli palatini).

■ PRIMARY TISSUES

Tissues are groups of cells with similar structure that perform a common function. The four primary tissue groups are as follows:
1. Epithelial
2. Connective
3. Muscular
4. Nervous

Epithelial Tissue (Epithelium, Epithelia)

Epithelia cover surfaces of the body and the body cavities of different systems (respiratory, digestive, cardiac, and vascular systems). This group of tissue performs the following functions:
• Protection
• Absorption and filtration
• Excretion and secretion
• Sensation

Connective Tissue

Connective tissue is a key component (with muscles and the skeleton) of the musculoskeletal system. It is widespread in the human body, and its principal functions are as follows:
• Fixation and support
• Protection
• Energy reserve
• Transportation of fluids and other substances
    Connective tissue can be solid, liquid, or gelatinous and can be classified in several different ways. The following four categories and respective subdivisions are used throughout the atlas: (1) connective tissue proper, (2) specialized connective tissues, (3) osseous tissue, and (4) blood.

Connective Tissue Proper

- **Loose (areolar)** connective tissue is a supple and gelatinous tissue formed of collagen and elastin fibers that surrounds and forms a cushion for organs and other body structures.
- **Adipose** connective tissue is composed of adipose cells and stores fat, protects and supports certain organs, and acts as an insulator.
- **Dense** connective tissue. Although the following classification system is often used, dense connective tissue types (together with elastic tissues) are more of a continuum than discrete entities.
  - **Dense regular** connective tissue is composed primarily of collagen fibers and some elastic fibers that follow a parallel orientation. It interconnects and supports body structures. Collagen fibers are quite stiff relative to elastic fibers and take longer to recover from deformation (like stretch). Tendons, ligaments, fascia, and aponeuroses (see next page) are composed of dense regular connective tissue.
  - **Dense irregular** connective tissue is principally composed of collagen fibers with no specific orientation. Its function is to reinforce and protect. Dense irregular connective tissue is found in the deep fascia of the body and the dermis (skin).
- **Elastic** connective tissue has a high concentration of elastic fibers (elastin and others), and this tissue recovers from deformation (stretch) very quickly like an elastic band. Such tissues are found in the bronchial tree and larynx including the vocal ligament of the vocal folds.

Specialized Connective Tissues

Cartilage (see Figure 3, p. 8)

- **Hyaline** cartilage is the most common cartilage. It contains collagen fibers and provides strength and flexibility. Some examples are costal, nasal, tracheal, and most laryngeal cartilages.
- **Elastic** cartilage is similar to hyaline cartilage but contains more elastic fibers and is thus more flexible. Some examples are the external ear, eustachian tube, epiglottis, cuneiform, and corniculate cartilages.
- **Fibrocartilage** is composed of dense collagen fibers and provides strength and shock absorption. Examples are the intervertebral discs.

More detail is provided on the following types of connective tissues that appear frequently in the atlas:

- **Membranes** are layers of epithelial and/or connective tissue that cover and protect body cavities and other surfaces. There are four types of membranes: mucous, serous, synovial, and cutaneous.
- **Tendons** are strong bands of dense regular connective tissue that connect skeletal muscle to bone. Tendons are flexible but resist extension (stretch). They are supplied with important sensory nerve endings, the Golgi tendon organs.
- **Aponeuroses** are broad tendinous-like sheets that cover muscle or are the points of origin or insertion of skeletal muscle.
- **Ligaments** are strong bands of dense regular connective tissue that connect bone to bone, cartilage to cartilage, and cartilage to bone. Ligaments are slightly elastic ("stretchy") and lengthen under tension.
- **Fascia** is connective tissue that covers and groups anatomical structures (muscles and organs) and also serves as a point of attachment of some muscles.

Osseous Tissue

Osseous tissue is hard and rigid tissue that is composed of collagen fibers and minerals. Bones produce red and white blood cells, store minerals, support the body, protect vital organs, and provide skeletal support for movement. They also serve a sound transmission role in bone-conducted hearing.

Blood

Although a fluid, blood is classified as a specialized connective tissue. It is composed of red blood cells, white blood cells, and platelets suspended in plasma. It transports respiratory gases, nutrients, and other substances crucial for normal body functions.

Muscular Tissue

- **Skeletal** muscles are composed of striated muscle fibers and are involved in the voluntary and involuntary control of body movements.
- **Cardiac** muscles are composed of striated cells and have involuntary control of the heart.
- **Smooth** muscles are composed of non-striated cells and are involved in the involuntary control of body organs.

Nervous Tissue

The nervous system is composed of the following types of nervous tissue:
- Neurons are specialized cells that conduct nerve impulses.
- Glial cells are non-conducting cells that support, insulate, and protect neurons.

■ TERMS RELATIVE TO BONES

Terms relative to bones are classified into the following categories:
1. Depressions
2. Elevations

Depressions

- A fissure is a cleft.
- A foramen is a natural opening (Figure 6; see also Figure 7, p. 18).
- A fossa is a depression (Figure 7, p. 18).
- A groove is a furrow.
- Meatus is a passageway (Figures 7 and 8, pp. 18 and 19).
- Sinus is a cavity (Figure 8, p. 19).

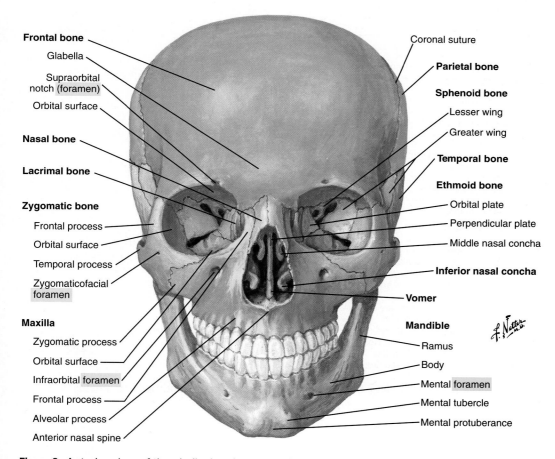

Figure 6. Anterior view of the skull, showing examples of the foramen, tubercle, and protuberance.

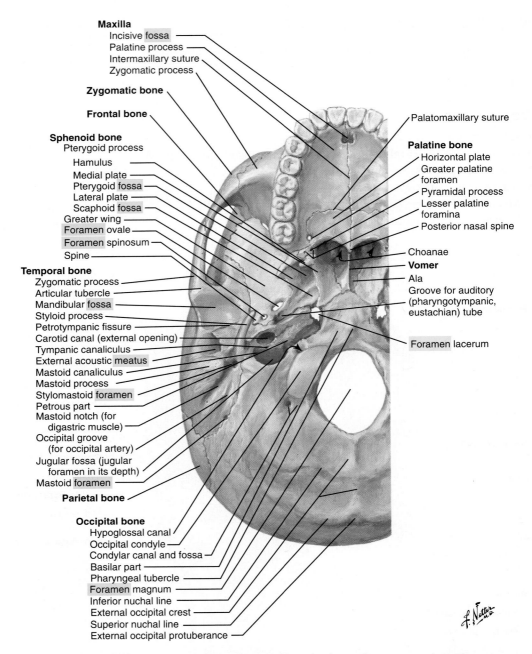

Maxilla
Incisive fossa
Palatine process
Intermaxillary suture
Zygomatic process

Zygomatic bone

Frontal bone

Sphenoid bone
Pterygoid process
Hamulus
Medial plate
Pterygoid fossa
Lateral plate
Scaphoid fossa
Greater wing
Foramen ovale
Foramen spinosum
Spine

Temporal bone
Zygomatic process
Articular tubercle
Mandibular fossa
Styloid process
Petrotympanic fissure
Carotid canal (external opening)
Tympanic canaliculus
External acoustic meatus
Mastoid canaliculus
Mastoid process
Stylomastoid foramen
Petrous part
Mastoid notch (for digastric muscle)
Occipital groove (for occipital artery)
Jugular fossa (jugular foramen in its depth)
Mastoid foramen

Parietal bone

Occipital bone
Hypoglossal canal
Occipital condyle
Condylar canal and fossa
Basilar part
Pharyngeal tubercle
Foramen magnum
Inferior nuchal line
External occipital crest
Superior nuchal line
External occipital protuberance

Palatomaxillary suture

Palatine bone
Horizontal plate
Greater palatine foramen
Pyramidal process
Lesser palatine foramina
Posterior nasal spine

Choanae

Vomer
Ala
Groove for auditory (pharyngotympanic, eustachian) tube

Foramen lacerum

Figure 7. Inferior view of the cranial base. Note the fossa, foramen, and meatus.

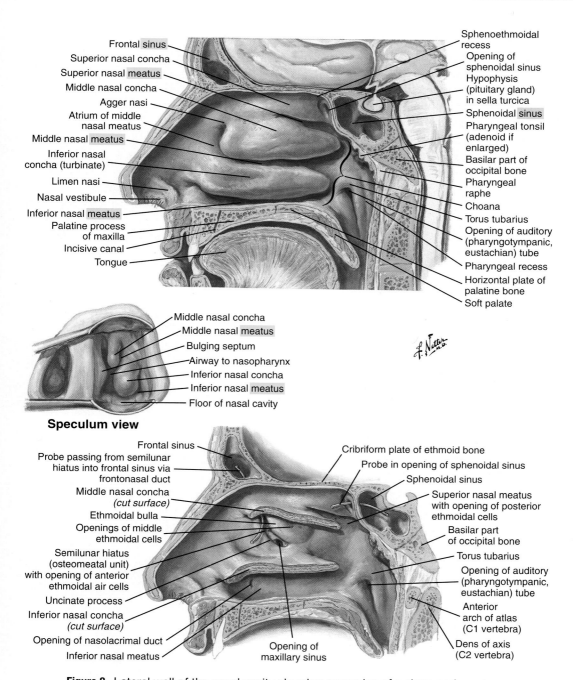

Frontal sinus
Superior nasal concha
Superior nasal meatus
Middle nasal concha
Agger nasi
Atrium of middle nasal meatus
Middle nasal meatus
Inferior nasal concha (turbinate)
Limen nasi
Nasal vestibule
Inferior nasal meatus
Palatine process of maxilla
Incisive canal
Tongue

Sphenoethmoidal recess
Opening of sphenoidal sinus
Hypophysis (pituitary gland) in sella turcica
Sphenoidal sinus
Pharyngeal tonsil (adenoid if enlarged)
Basilar part of occipital bone
Pharyngeal raphe
Choana
Torus tubarius
Opening of auditory (pharyngotympanic, eustachian) tube
Pharyngeal recess
Horizontal plate of palatine bone
Soft palate

Middle nasal concha
Middle nasal meatus
Bulging septum
Airway to nasopharynx
Inferior nasal concha
Inferior nasal meatus
Floor of nasal cavity

Speculum view

Frontal sinus
Probe passing from semilunar hiatus into frontal sinus via frontonasal duct
Middle nasal concha (cut surface)
Ethmoidal bulla
Openings of middle ethmoidal cells
Semilunar hiatus (osteomeatal unit) with opening of anterior ethmoidal air cells
Uncinate process
Inferior nasal concha (cut surface)
Opening of nasolacrimal duct
Inferior nasal meatus

Cribriform plate of ethmoid bone
Probe in opening of sphenoidal sinus
Sphenoidal sinus
Superior nasal meatus with opening of posterior ethmoidal cells
Basilar part of occipital bone
Torus tubarius
Opening of auditory (pharyngotympanic, eustachian) tube
Anterior arch of atlas (C1 vertebra)
Dens of axis (C2 vertebra)

Opening of maxillary sinus

Figure 8. Lateral wall of the nasal cavity showing examples of a sinus and meatus.

Elevations

- Condyle is a rounded point of articulation (Figure 9).
- Crest is a ridge (see Figure 9).
- Head is an enlargement of the extremity of a bone (see Figure 9).
- Process is a prominence or extension (see also Figure 7, p. 18).
- Protuberance is a projection beyond the surface.
- Spine is a spike-shaped projection.
- Tubercle is a small, rounded protuberance (see Figure 9; see also Figure 6, p. 17).
- Tuberosity is a larger, rounded protuberance (see Figure 9).

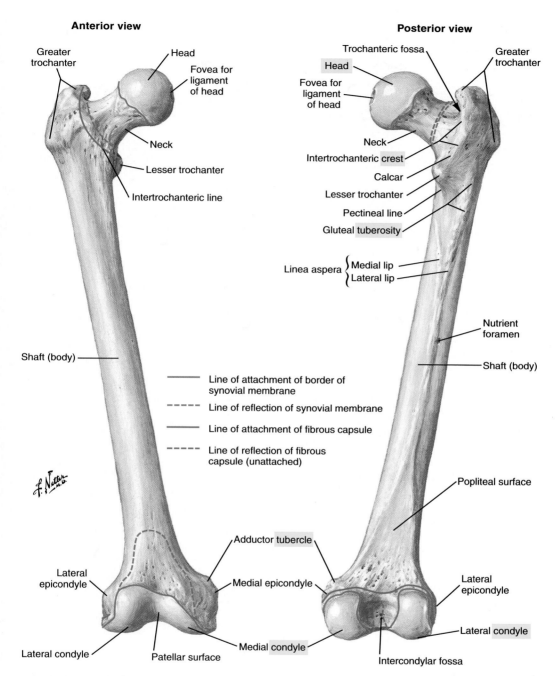

Anterior view

Greater trochanter

Head

Fovea for ligament of head

Neck

Lesser trochanter

Intertrochanteric line

Shaft (body)

——— Line of attachment of border of synovial membrane

- - - - - Line of reflection of synovial membrane

——— Line of attachment of fibrous capsule

- - - - - Line of reflection of fibrous capsule (unattached)

Lateral epicondyle

Lateral condyle

Patellar surface

Adductor tubercle

Medial epicondyle

Medial condyle

Posterior view

Trochanteric fossa

Head

Fovea for ligament of head

Neck

Intertrochanteric crest

Calcar

Lesser trochanter

Pectineal line

Gluteal tuberosity

Linea aspera { Medial lip
Lateral lip

Greater trochanter

Nutrient foramen

Shaft (body)

Popliteal surface

Lateral epicondyle

Lateral condyle

Intercondylar fossa

Figure 9. Anterior and posterior views of the femur. Note the condyle, crest, head, tubercle, and tuberosity.

RESPIRATORY SYSTEM

1

■ OVERVIEW

The respiratory system is vital for the elimination of carbon dioxide and the absorption of oxygen. Superimposed on this primary biological function is the use of the respiratory system for speech production. The respiratory system is the source of energy for vocal fold vibration and consonant production by the oral articulators.

For speech production, the pressure beneath the closed vocal folds (subglottal pressure) is maintained within a relatively narrow range. The maintenance of a relatively constant subglottal pressure requires a complex interaction between the forces generated by the passive mechanical properties of the lungs and thorax and those generated by active muscular contraction. Even though subglottal pressure is maintained relatively constant for vocal fold vibration, it is possible to modulate this pressure up or down for changes in loudness (intensity) or pitch (fundamental frequency).

Inspirations during speech are rapid to avoid interruptions to the flow of speech and terminate at slightly higher lung volumes than those associated with quiet breathing. Expirations are prolonged, and because we speak during the expiratory phase, their duration is influenced by communication demands.

For swallowing, the precise coordination of respiratory and swallowing processes ensures adequate airway protection. The airway is protected during swallowing because the food or liquid bolus and air share a common passageway and aspiration must be prevented. Airway protective mechanisms during swallowing include respiratory inhibition, vocal fold closure, laryngeal elevation, and velopharyngeal closure.

The respiratory system is the topic of Part 1, beginning with a brief overview of the skeletal support for respiration and then addressing the lungs and associated respiratory structures. Finally, respiratory muscles and their functions are reviewed.

■ SKELETAL SUPPORT FOR RESPIRATION

Skeletal support for respiration is composed of the following elements (see Figures 1-3 and 1-4, pp. 31 and 33):
- Posteriorly by the vertebral column
- Anteriorly by the sternum and cartilages
- Laterally by the ribs
- Superiorly by the scapular girdle
- Inferiorly by the pelvic girdle

Vertebral Column (Figure 1-1)

The vertebral column contains 32 to 33 vertebrae that are numbered superiorly to inferiorly in five regions, as follows:
- 7 cervical vertebrae
- 12 thoracic vertebrae (that articulate with 12 ribs)
- 5 lumbar vertebrae
- 5 sacral vertebrae
- 3 to 4 coccygeal vertebrae

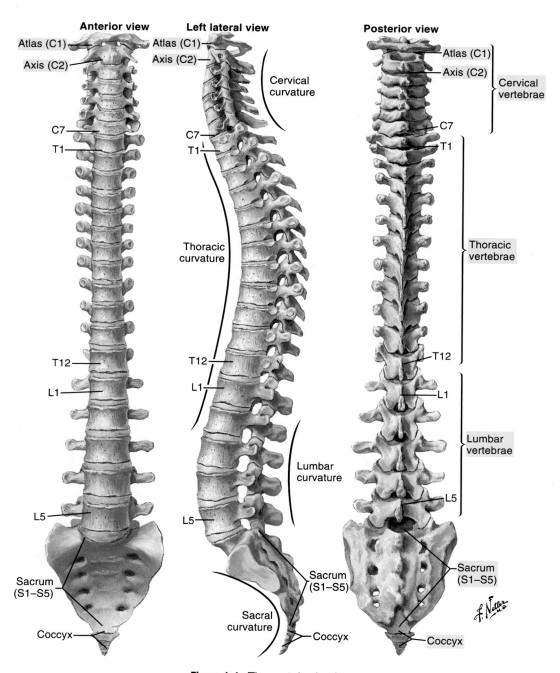

Anterior view

Atlas (C1)
Axis (C2)

C7
T1

T12

L1

L5

Sacrum
(S1–S5)

Coccyx

Left lateral view

Atlas (C1)
Axis (C2)

Cervical
curvature

C7
T1

Thoracic
curvature

T12

L1

Lumbar
curvature

L5

Sacrum
(S1–S5)

Sacral
curvature

Coccyx

Posterior view

Atlas (C1)
Axis (C2)

Cervical
vertebrae

C7

T1

Thoracic
vertebrae

T12

L1

Lumbar
vertebrae

L5

Sacrum
(S1–S5)

Coccyx

Figure 1-1. The vertebral column.

A typical thoracic vertebra contains the following elements (Figure 1-2):
- Vertebral body
- Vertebral foramen (canal for the spinal cord)
- Four articular processes where adjacent vertebrae connect (to *articulate* means to "come closer and form a junction")
- Superior and transverse costal facets, which are points of attachment of the ribs
- Transverse processes, which are points of attachment of muscles and ligaments
- A spinous process, which is the site of attachment of muscles and ligaments
  Refer to Figure 1-1 (p. 27) to see the following:
- Note the change in the form of the vertebrae. Inferior vertebrae are more massive to support more weight.
- The vertebral column contains four curves (cervical, thoracic, lumbar, and sacral). These curves give a double S shape to the vertebral column and increase its strength and flexibility to support body weight and movement.
- Two cervical vertebrae have anatomical and functional characteristics that are different from the other vertebrae. The first cervical vertebra (C1), or atlas (after Greek mythology), has no body or spinous process, supports the head, and allows for head rotation and other movements. The second cervical vertebra (C2), or axis, has an odontoid (meaning toothlike) process that serves as a pivot point for head rotation.
- The seventh cervical vertebra (C7) has a long spinous process that is often easy to locate and palpate on the skin's surface.
- Sacral vertebrae are normally fused in the adult. They reinforce and stabilize the pelvis and form the sacrum.
- Coccygeal vertebrae are also fused and form a small triangular bone, the coccyx.
- Intervertebral discs of fibrocartilage lie between adjacent vertebrae except for between the atlas and axis and in between adjacent sacral and coccygeal vertebrae (which are fused). There is a large intervertebral disc between the last lumbar (L5) and first sacral (S1) vertebrae (the lumbosacral joint) and a small atypical disc between the last sacral (S5) and first coccygeal (Co1) vertebrae (the sacrococcygeal joint). Discs provide for movement and shock absorption.

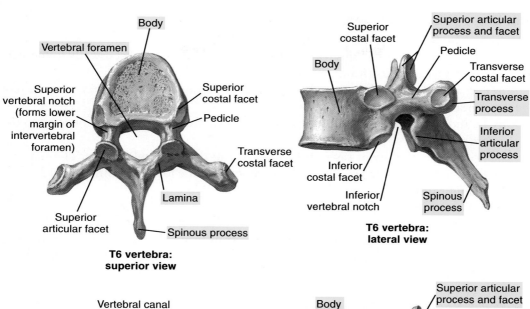

T6 vertebra: superior view

Body

Vertebral foramen

Superior vertebral notch (forms lower margin of intervertebral foramen)

Superior costal facet

Pedicle

Superior articular facet

Lamina

Spinous process

Transverse costal facet

T6 vertebra: lateral view

Superior costal facet

Superior articular process and facet

Pedicle

Transverse costal facet

Transverse process

Body

Inferior articular process

Inferior costal facet

Inferior vertebral notch

Spinous process

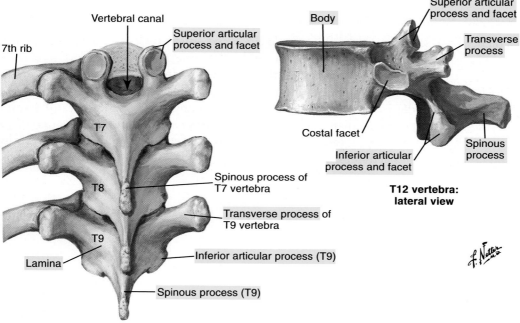

T7, T8, and T9 vertebrae: posterior view

Vertebral canal

Superior articular process and facet

7th rib

T7

T8

T9

Lamina

Spinous process of T7 vertebra

Transverse process of T9 vertebra

Inferior articular process (T9)

Spinous process (T9)

T12 vertebra: lateral view

Body

Superior articular process and facet

Transverse process

Costal facet

Inferior articular process and facet

Spinous process

Figure 1-2. The thoracic vertebrae.

Rib Cage (Ribs, Cartilages, Sternum) (Figure 1-3)

The human body contains the following 12 pairs of ribs:

- Ribs 1 through 7 are "true" ribs (or vertebrosternal ribs) and connect directly to the sternum via costal cartilages (for mobility).
- Ribs 8, 9, and 10 are "false" ribs and connect to the sternum via a common cartilage that joins the seventh costal cartilage.
- Ribs 11 and 12 are "floating" ribs; their anterior extremity is free (not connected to the sternum).

The posterior extremity of each rib is connected to the vertebral column. The sternum is connected to the ribs and clavicles and is composed of the following three parts:

1. The manubrium
2. The body or corpus
3. The xiphoid process

The articulation of the manubrium with the corpus forms the sternal angle, or angle of Louis, and marks the approximate location of the second costal cartilages and the level of tracheal bifurcation.

Pectoral, Scapular, or Shoulder Girdle (see Figure 1-3)

- The pectoral, scapular, or shoulder girdle is formed anteriorly by the clavicle (long thin bone) and posteriorly by the scapula (triangular flat bone).
- The clavicle allows for the projection of the scapula away from the thoracic cage.
- The humerus is attached to the glenoid fossa of the scapula.
- The pectoral girdle is the point of attachment for many accessory muscles of respiration such as the pectoralis major and subclavian muscles. Fixation or stabilization of the pectoral girdle is needed for forced inspiration and expiration, as well as for heavy lifting and other strenuous activities.

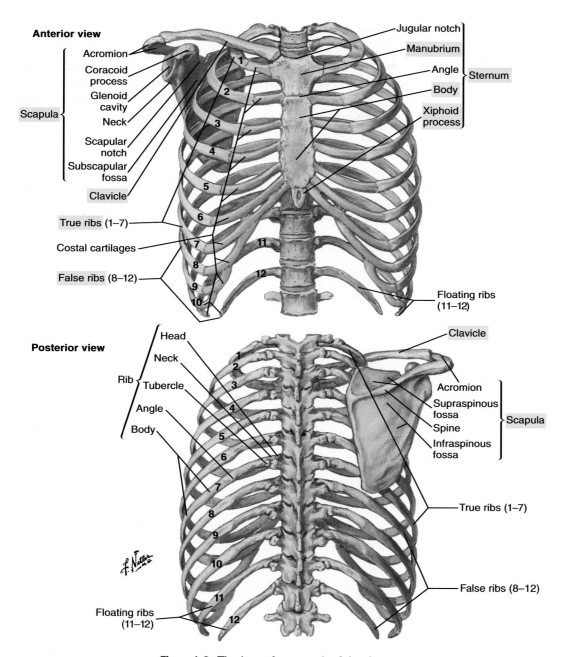

Figure 1-3. The bony framework of the thorax.

Pelvic Girdle or Bony Pelvis (Figure 1-4)

The pelvic girdle is formed by the following:

- A pair of symmetrical coxal, or hip, bones that are joined together anteriorly at the pubic symphysis and posteriorly by the sacrum. Each hip bone is composed of three distinct bones that fuse during development. The following individual structures retain their names despite the fact that they are fused and no suture lines may visible:
  - Ilium
  - Ischium
  - Pubis
- The sacrum is attached to the ilium at the sacroiliac joint, an extremely strong and stable joint that supports the weight of the upper body.
- The coccyx is the final segment of the vertebral column and is often referred to as the "tailbone."

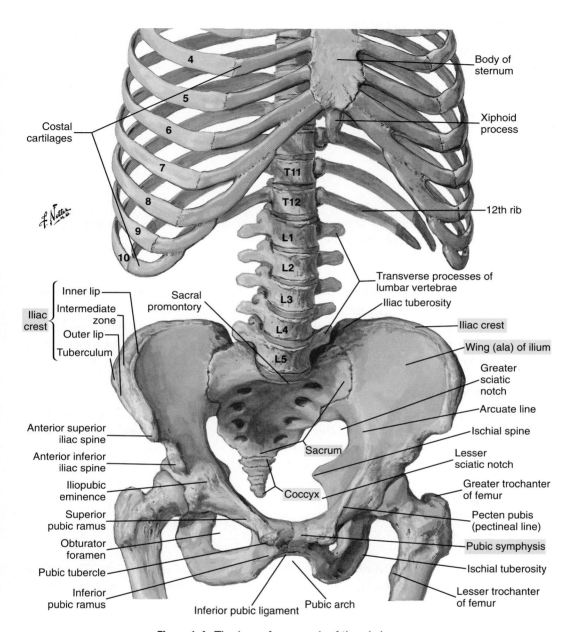

Body of sternum

Xiphoid process

Costal cartilages

4
5
6
7
8
9
10

T11
T12

12th rib

L1
L2

Transverse processes of lumbar vertebrae

Iliac crest
Inner lip
Intermediate zone
Outer lip
Tuberculum

Sacral promontory

L3
L4
L5

Iliac tuberosity
Iliac crest
Wing (ala) of ilium
Greater sciatic notch
Arcuate line
Ischial spine

Anterior superior iliac spine

Anterior inferior iliac spine

Sacrum

Lesser sciatic notch

Greater trochanter of femur

Iliopubic eminence

Superior pubic ramus

Obturator foramen

Pubic tubercle

Inferior pubic ramus

Coccyx

Pecten pubis (pectineal line)
Pubic symphysis
Ischial tuberosity
Lesser trochanter of femur

Inferior pubic ligament   Pubic arch

Figure 1-4. The bony framework of the abdomen.

■ RESPIRATORY TRACT

Air circulates in the following respiratory areas:
- Nasal cavities
- Oral cavity
- Pharynx
- Larynx
- Trachea
- Bronchi
- Lungs

Nasal Cavities (Figure 1-5)

The nasal cavities are the first segment of the upper respiratory tract and participate in olfaction (see Part 3: Articulatory System, pp. 105–167).

Oral Cavity

The oral cavity is delimited anteriorly and laterally by the teeth, posteriorly by the palatoglossal arch (anterior faucial pillar), superiorly by the hard palate and soft palate, and inferiorly by the tongue. It is located behind and medial to the buccal cavity, which is the space between the lips and gums and the teeth, and anterior to the pharynx (see Part 3: Articulatory System, pp. 105–167).

Pharynx (Figure 1-6, p. 36)

The pharynx is a vertically oriented muscular passageway that provides communication between the buccal/oral cavities and the esophagus and between the nasal cavities and the larynx (see Part 3: Articulatory System, pp. 105–167).

The pharynx is composed of the following:
- Nasal portion (nasopharynx)
- Buccal portion (oropharynx)
- Laryngeal portion (laryngopharynx)

Larynx (Figure 1-7, p. 37)

The larynx is located directly above the trachea and in front of the pharynx. The principal biological function of the larynx is to protect the lower respiratory tract (see Part 2: Phonatory System, pp. 73–103).

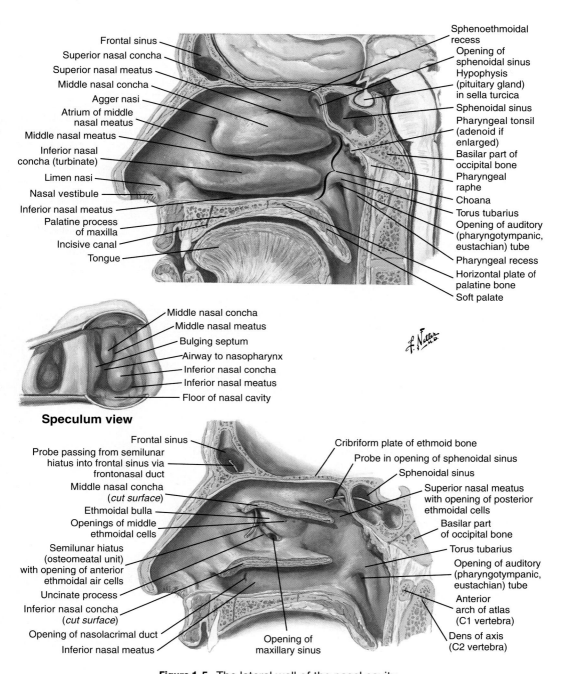

Frontal sinus
Superior nasal concha
Superior nasal meatus
Middle nasal concha
Agger nasi
Atrium of middle
nasal meatus
Middle nasal meatus
Inferior nasal
concha (turbinate)
Limen nasi
Nasal vestibule
Inferior nasal meatus
Palatine process
of maxilla
Incisive canal
Tongue

Sphenoethmoidal
recess
Opening of
sphenoidal sinus
Hypophysis
(pituitary gland)
in sella turcica
Sphenoidal sinus
Pharyngeal tonsil
(adenoid if
enlarged)
Basilar part of
occipital bone
Pharyngeal
raphe
Choana
Torus tubarius
Opening of auditory
(pharyngotympanic,
eustachian) tube
Pharyngeal recess
Horizontal plate of
palatine bone
Soft palate

Middle nasal concha
Middle nasal meatus
Bulging septum
Airway to nasopharynx
Inferior nasal concha
Inferior nasal meatus
Floor of nasal cavity

Speculum view

Frontal sinus
Probe passing from semilunar
hiatus into frontal sinus via
frontonasal duct
Middle nasal concha
(*cut surface*)
Ethmoidal bulla
Openings of middle
ethmoidal cells
Semilunar hiatus
(osteomeatal unit)
with opening of anterior
ethmoidal air cells
Uncinate process
Inferior nasal concha
(*cut surface*)
Opening of nasolacrimal duct
Inferior nasal meatus

Cribriform plate of ethmoid bone
Probe in opening of sphenoidal sinus
Sphenoidal sinus
Superior nasal meatus
with opening of posterior
ethmoidal cells
Basilar part
of occipital bone
Torus tubarius
Opening of auditory
(pharyngotympanic,
eustachian) tube
Anterior
arch of atlas
(C1 vertebra)
Dens of axis
(C2 vertebra)

Opening of
maxillary sinus

Figure 1-5. The lateral wall of the nasal cavity.

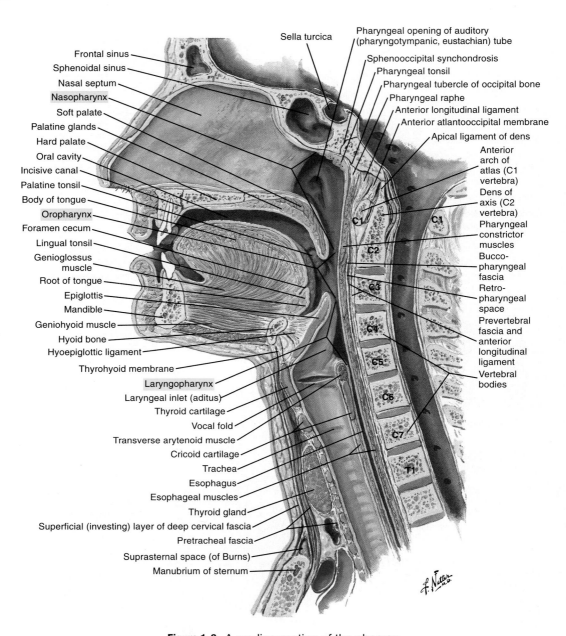

Sella turcica

Pharyngeal opening of auditory
(pharyngotympanic, eustachian) tube

Frontal sinus

Sphenoidal sinus

Nasal septum

Nasopharynx

Soft palate

Palatine glands

Hard palate

Oral cavity

Incisive canal

Palatine tonsil

Body of tongue

Oropharynx

Foramen cecum

Lingual tonsil

Genioglossus
muscle

Root of tongue

Epiglottis

Mandible

Geniohyoid muscle

Hyoid bone

Hyoepiglottic ligament

Thyrohyoid membrane

Laryngopharynx

Laryngeal inlet (aditus)

Thyroid cartilage

Vocal fold

Transverse arytenoid muscle

Cricoid cartilage

Trachea

Esophagus

Esophageal muscles

Thyroid gland

Superficial (investing) layer of deep cervical fascia

Pretracheal fascia

Suprasternal space (of Burns)

Manubrium of sternum

Sphenooccipital synchondrosis

Pharyngeal tonsil

Pharyngeal tubercle of occipital bone

Pharyngeal raphe

Anterior longitudinal ligament

Anterior atlantooccipital membrane

Apical ligament of dens

Anterior
arch of
atlas (C1
vertebra)

Dens of
axis (C2
vertebra)

Pharyngeal
constrictor
muscles

Bucco-
pharyngeal
fascia

Retro-
pharyngeal
space

Prevertebral
fascia and
anterior
longitudinal
ligament

Vertebral
bodies

Figure 1-6. A median section of the pharynx.

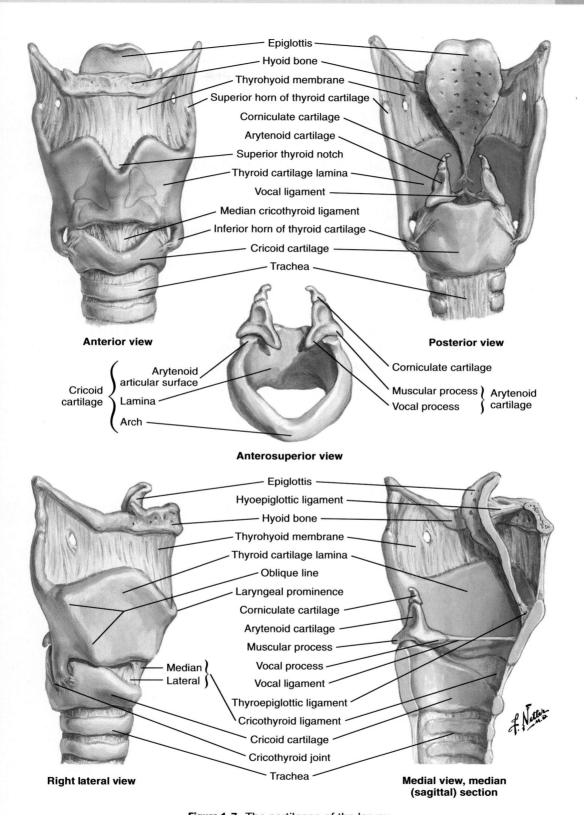

Epiglottis

Hyoid bone

Thyrohyoid membrane

Superior horn of thyroid cartilage

Corniculate cartilage

Arytenoid cartilage

Superior thyroid notch

Thyroid cartilage lamina

Vocal ligament

Median cricothyroid ligament

Inferior horn of thyroid cartilage

Cricoid cartilage

Trachea

Anterior view

Posterior view

Arytenoid articular surface

Cricoid cartilage

Lamina

Arch

Corniculate cartilage

Muscular process } Arytenoid cartilage

Vocal process

Anterosuperior view

Epiglottis

Hyoepiglottic ligament

Hyoid bone

Thyrohyoid membrane

Thyroid cartilage lamina

Oblique line

Laryngeal prominence

Corniculate cartilage

Arytenoid cartilage

Muscular process

Median }
Lateral }

Vocal process

Vocal ligament

Thyroepiglottic ligament

Cricothyroid ligament

Cricoid cartilage

Cricothyroid joint

Trachea

Right lateral view

Medial view, median (sagittal) section

Figure 1-7. The cartilages of the larynx.

Trachea (Figure 1-8)

The trachea extends from the larynx to the bronchi. It contains 16 to 20 incomplete cartilaginous horseshoe-shaped rings connected by membranes. The rings are deficient posteriorly to accommodate the attachment to the esophagus. The trachea has two portions: (1) cervical and (2) thoracic.

Bronchi (Figures 1-8 and 1-9 [p. 40])

The trachea divides, or bifurcates, at the level of the sternal angle (T4 to T5) to form the main, or primary, bronchi (right and left), as follows:

- The main bronchi divide into lobar or secondary bronchi: one for each lung lobe, three for the right (superior, middle, and inferior), and two for the left (superior and inferior).
- The lobar bronchi further divide to form segmental or tertiary bronchi (third-order bronchi): each supplying a specific bronchopulmonary segment, 10 for the right, and 9 for the left.
- The segmental bronchi continue to divide many times (20 to 25 generations) to eventually become terminal bronchioles ("little tubes") with diameters of less than 0.5 mm. The terminal bronchioles are the end of the conducting respiratory passageways.

The respiratory portion of the pathway in which gas exchange occurs begins with the respiratory bronchioles, then the alveolar ducts, the alveolar sacs, and the alveoli, in which the main part of pulmonary gas exchange occurs (Figure 1-10, p. 41).

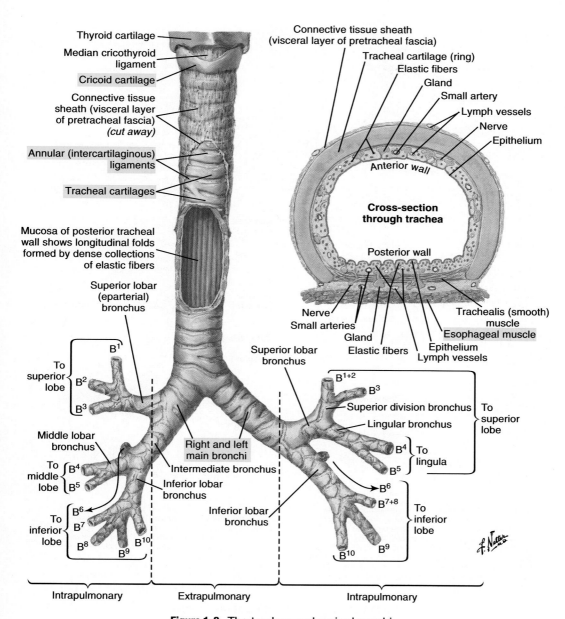

Figure 1-8. The trachea and major bronchi.

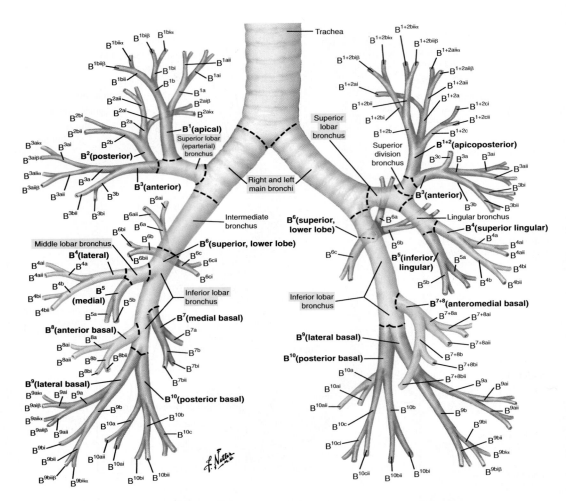

Trachea

B^{1}(apical)
Superior lobar
(eparterial)
bronchus

B^{2}(posterior)

B^{3}(anterior)

Superior
lobar
bronchus

Superior
division
bronchus

B^{1+2}(apicoposterior)

B^{3}(anterior)

Right and left
main bronchi

Intermediate
bronchus

B^{6}(superior,
lower lobe)

Lingular bronchus

B^{4}(superior lingular)

B^{6}(superior, lower lobe)

Middle lobar bronchus

B^{4}(lateral)

B^{5}(inferior,
lingular)

B^{5}
(medial)

Inferior lobar
bronchus

B^{7}(medial basal)

Inferior lobar
bronchus

B^{7+8}(anteromedial basal)

B^{8}(anterior basal)

B^{9}(lateral basal)

B^{10}(posterior basal)

B^{9}(lateral basal)

B^{10}(posterior basal)

Nomenclature in common usage for bronchopulmonary
segments is that of Jackson and Huber, and segmental
bronchi are named accordingly. Ikeda proposed
nomenclature (as demonstrated here) for bronchial
subdivisions as far as 6th generation. For simplification on
this illustration, only some bronchial subdivisions are labeled
as far as 5th or 6th generation. Segmental bronchi (B) are
numbered from 1 to 10 in each lung, corresponding to
pulmonary segments. In left lung,

B^{1} and B^{2} are combined, as are B^{7} and B^{8}. Subsegmental,
or 4th order, bronchi are indicated by addition of lower-
case letters a, b, or c when an additional branch is present.
Fifth order bronchi are designated by Roman numerals i
(anterior) or ii (posterior) and 6th order bronchi by Greek
letters α or β. Several texts use alternate numbers (as
proposed by Boyden) for segmental bronchi.
    Variations of standard bronchial pattern shown here
are common, especially in peripheral airways.

Figure 1-9. The nomenclature of the bronchi.

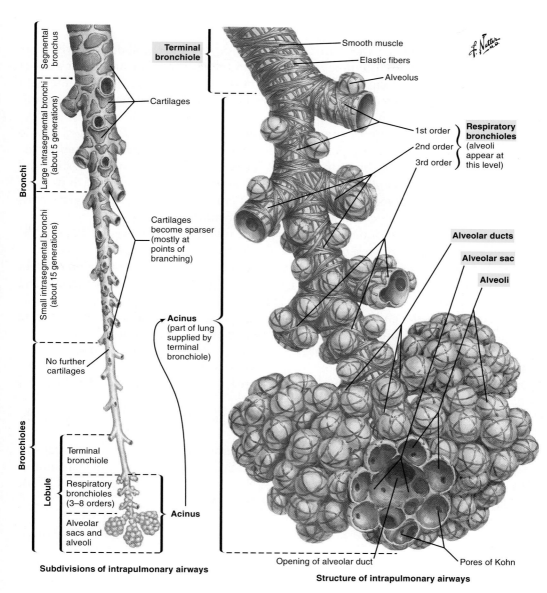

Subdivisions of intrapulmonary airways

Structure of intrapulmonary airways

Figure 1-10. The intrapulmonary airways. Gas exchange begins at the level of the respiratory bronchioles.

Lungs (Figure 1-11)

The trunk, or torso, contains the thorax (or thoracic cavity) and the abdomen, which are divided by the diaphragm. The lungs are located in the thorax. They are two masses of nonmuscular tissue that occupy a major portion of the thoracic cavity. Between the right and left lungs is a space called the *mediastinum* that contains the heart and other anatomical structures (Figure 1-12, p. 44).

The lungs are spongy, porous, and highly elastic. Because they are elastic, they seek to return to their relaxed or resting position when stretched or compressed and can generate relaxation pressures because of their elastic recoil. Imagine stretching an elastic band between your two fingers and "feeling" the tension acting to return the band to its non-stretched position. Elastic recoil forces of the lungs (and thorax) and the pulmonary pressures they create are key aspects of quiet and speech breathing.

Although similar in appearance and function, the following differences in shape of the two lungs are a result of the presence of adjacent organs (Figure 1-13, p. 45):

- The right lung is larger and broader than the left but shorter because of the presence of the liver and the elevation of the diaphragm on the right side. The overall capacity and weight of the right lung is greater than the left.
- The left lung is smaller and narrower than the right lung, with a distinct cardiac notch to accommodate the pericardium (containing the heart and other great blood vessels).
- The right lung is divided into three lobes by the horizontal and oblique fissures.
- The left lung is divided into two lobes by an oblique fissure.
- Each lung is anatomically divided into functional segments called *bronchopulmonary segments* (10 for the right and 9 for the left).
- The superior aspect of each lung is called the *apex,* and the inferior aspect is called the *base.*
- Each lung has an inferior concave diaphragmatic surface, an external convex costal surface, and an internal concave surface that is caused by the presence of the mediastinum.
- The lung apex can exceed the limits of the thorax and protrude above the level of the middle third of the clavicle by several centimeters.

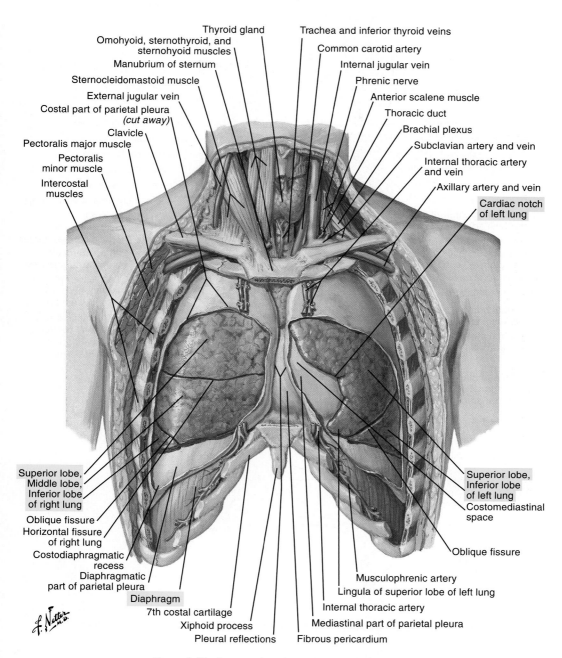

Thyroid gland

Omohyoid, sternothyroid, and
sternohyoid muscles

Manubrium of sternum

Sternocleidomastoid muscle

External jugular vein

Costal part of parietal pleura
(cut away)

Clavicle

Pectoralis major muscle

Pectoralis
minor muscle

Intercostal
muscles

Trachea and inferior thyroid veins

Common carotid artery

Internal jugular vein

Phrenic nerve

Anterior scalene muscle

Thoracic duct

Brachial plexus

Subclavian artery and vein

Internal thoracic artery
and vein

Axillary artery and vein

Cardiac notch
of left lung

Superior lobe,
Middle lobe,
Inferior lobe
of right lung

Oblique fissure

Horizontal fissure
of right lung

Costodiaphragmatic
recess

Diaphragmatic
part of parietal pleura

Diaphragm

7th costal cartilage

Xiphoid process

Pleural reflections

Superior lobe,
Inferior lobe
of left lung

Costomediastinal
space

Oblique fissure

Musculophrenic artery

Lingula of superior lobe of left lung

Internal thoracic artery

Mediastinal part of parietal pleura

Fibrous pericardium

Figure 1-11. An anterior view of the lungs in situ.

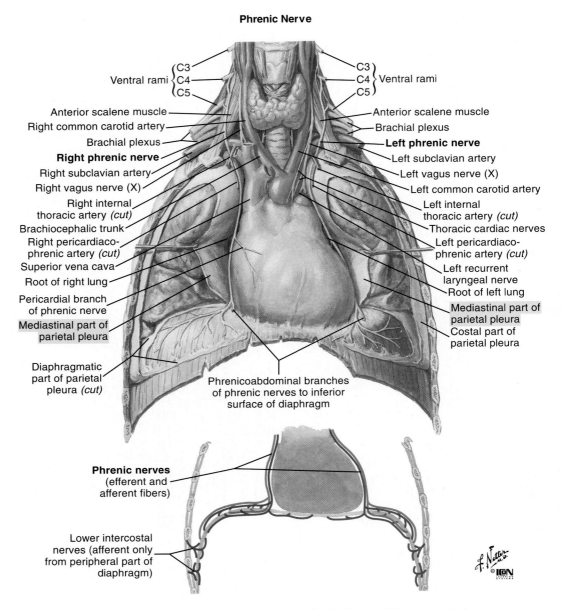

Figure 1-12. The phrenic nerve. Note the mediastinal part of the parietal pleura.

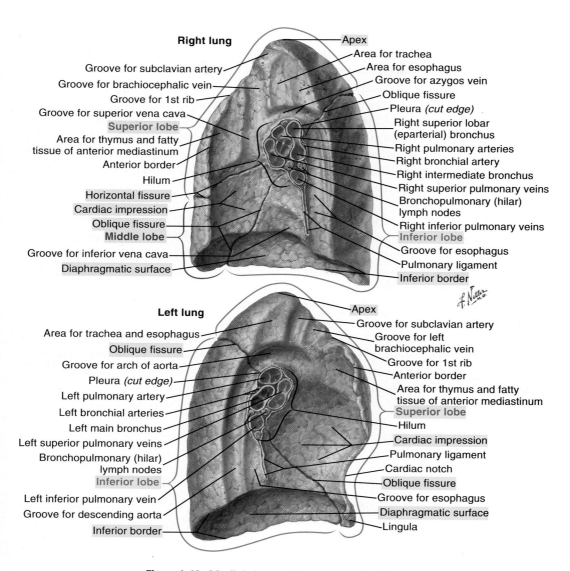

Right lung

Groove for subclavian artery
Groove for brachiocephalic vein
Groove for 1st rib
Groove for superior vena cava
Superior lobe
Area for thymus and fatty tissue of anterior mediastinum
Anterior border
Hilum
Horizontal fissure
Cardiac impression
Oblique fissure
Middle lobe
Groove for inferior vena cava
Diaphragmatic surface

Apex
Area for trachea
Area for esophagus
Groove for azygos vein
Oblique fissure
Pleura (cut edge)
Right superior lobar (eparterial) bronchus
Right pulmonary arteries
Right bronchial artery
Right intermediate bronchus
Right superior pulmonary veins
Bronchopulmonary (hilar) lymph nodes
Right inferior pulmonary veins
Inferior lobe
Groove for esophagus
Pulmonary ligament
Inferior border

Left lung

Area for trachea and esophagus
Oblique fissure
Groove for arch of aorta
Pleura (cut edge)
Left pulmonary artery
Left bronchial arteries
Left main bronchus
Left superior pulmonary veins
Bronchopulmonary (hilar) lymph nodes
Inferior lobe
Left inferior pulmonary vein
Groove for descending aorta
Inferior border

Apex
Groove for subclavian artery
Groove for left brachiocephalic vein
Groove for 1st rib
Anterior border
Area for thymus and fatty tissue of anterior mediastinum
Superior lobe
Hilum
Cardiac impression
Pulmonary ligament
Cardiac notch
Oblique fissure
Groove for esophagus
Diaphragmatic surface
Lingula

Figure 1-13. Medial views of the right and left lungs.

Pleura (Figure 1-14)

The pleurae are intrathoracic serous membranes that envelop and protect the lungs:
- The parietal pleurae line the inner surface of the thoracic cavity.
- The visceral pleurae cover each lung independently.

Parietal and visceral pleurae are attached (linked) through a very thin, fluid-filled space called the *pleural space*. Fluid in the space allows for friction-free movement between the two membranes and creates surface tension and negative pressure that link the two pleurae. With pleural linkage, when respiratory muscles change the dimensions of the thorax, lung volume also changes. Consequently, the lungs and thorax normally act as a unit and are often referred to as the *lungs-thorax unit*.

Selected Pulmonary Disorders Affecting Lung Function

- **Pleurisy** is an inflammation of the pleura caused by an undersecretion or oversecretion of fluid in the pleural space. Respiration may be very painful.
- **Pneumothorax** is the presence of air in the pleural space (the result of trauma such as a penetrating chest wound or disease). This condition may interrupt pleural linkage and cause a collapse of one or both of the lungs, depending on whether the pneumothorax is unilateral or bilateral.
- **Pneumonia** is an infection of the lungs resulting from many possible causes, including the presence of bacteria, viruses, and fungi. Pneumonia is a common consequence of disordered swallowing and the aspiration (breathing in) of food and liquids. This is referred to as *aspiration pneumonia*.

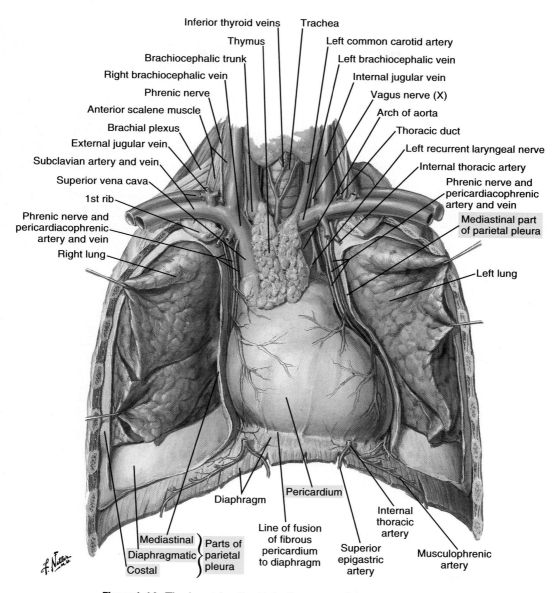

Inferior thyroid veins
Trachea
Thymus
Left common carotid artery
Brachiocephalic trunk
Left brachiocephalic vein
Right brachiocephalic vein
Internal jugular vein
Phrenic nerve
Vagus nerve (X)
Anterior scalene muscle
Arch of aorta
Brachial plexus
Thoracic duct
External jugular vein
Left recurrent laryngeal nerve
Subclavian artery and vein
Internal thoracic artery
Superior vena cava
Phrenic nerve and
pericardiacophrenic
artery and vein
1st rib
Phrenic nerve and
pericardiacophrenic
artery and vein
Mediastinal part
of parietal pleura
Right lung
Left lung
Diaphragm
Pericardium
Mediastinal
Diaphragmatic
Costal
Parts of parietal pleura
Line of fusion
of fibrous
pericardium
to diaphragm
Internal
thoracic
artery
Superior
epigastric
artery
Musculophrenic
artery

Figure 1-14. The heart in situ. Note the parts of the parietal pleura.

■ RESPIRATORY MUSCLES

A very large number of muscles are potentially involved in respiration. Our focus here is on the principal muscles of respiration, which are classified as either inspiratory or expiratory (see the tables on pp. 63, 64, and 67). This historical classification is based on the isolated action of each muscle. Inspiratory muscles are those muscles whose mechanical advantage or action is to increase lung volume, and expiratory muscles are those whose mechanical advantage or action is to decrease lung volume. However, it is important to note that inspiratory muscles are not solely active during inspiration, and expiratory muscles are not solely active during expiration. For example, during normal spontaneous breathing, the diaphragm (a major muscle of inspiration) continues to contract during the early expiratory phase to slow passive relaxation forces acting to decrease lung volume.

Therefore the muscles grouped in the category "inspiratory muscles" are those whose isolated action is to increase lung volume, and "expiratory muscles" are those whose isolated action is to decrease lung volume.

Principal Muscles of Inspiration

The function of the principal muscles of inspiration is to increase pulmonary volume.

Diaphragm (Figures 1-15 and 1-16, pp. 50 and 51)

The diaphragm is an unpaired muscle. It is a thin, dome-shaped muscle with a strong central tendon (aponeurosis). It separates the thorax from the abdomen. Several important structures pass through the diaphragm including the esophagus, aorta, and major veins through the following:

- Aortic hiatus
- Esophageal hiatus
- Vena cava foramen (caval opening)

The three main groups of muscle fibers, named according to their principal points of origin, are as follows:

1. The **costal part** originates from the inferior and inner surfaces of the costal cartilages and adjacent portions of the last six ribs and courses directly upward to insert into the central tendon. Costal diaphragm muscle fibers are directly apposed to the inner surface of the rib cage for approximately 6 to 9 cm through the "zone of apposition."

2. The **sternal part** originates from the inner inferior surface of the xiphoid process of the sternum and courses upward to insert into the central tendon.

3. The **lumbar** (vertebral) part originates from the upper lumbar vertebrae through two groups of fibers called *crura* and from the medial and lateral arcuate ligaments. Fibers course upward to insert into the central tendon.

The orientation of the fibers of the diaphragm can be visualized by imagining the fibers forming the inner walls of a bowl.

Diaphragm contraction (and shortening of its muscle fibers) pulls down on the central tendon, which increases the vertical dimensions of the lungs-thorax unit. At the level of the rib cage, diaphragm contraction (against the resistance of the abdominal contents) lifts the ribs and rotates them outward, which increases the anterolateral dimensions of the rib cage. Lung volume increases, thus creating negative (inspiratory) alveolar (lung) pressure. The contraction of the diaphragm compresses the viscera and increases abdominal pressure.

When the diaphragm relaxes, it returns to its resting form, thus decreasing the vertical dimensions of the lungs-thorax unit. The ribs also rotate downward and inward, decreasing circumferential dimensions.

The diaphragm is innervated by the phrenic nerve, which arises from cervical spinal nerves C3 to C5.

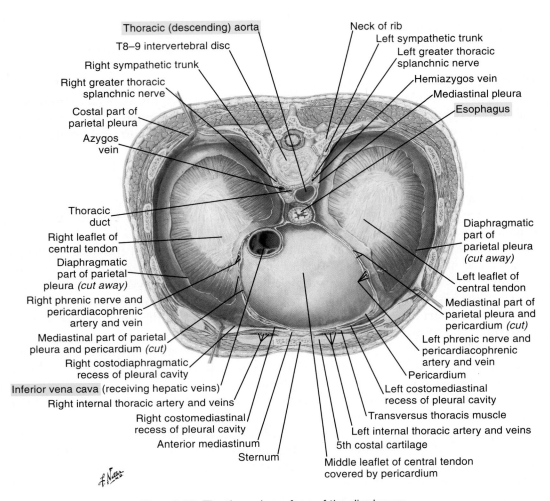

Thoracic (descending) aorta

Neck of rib

Left sympathetic trunk

T8–9 intervertebral disc

Left greater thoracic splanchnic nerve

Right sympathetic trunk

Hemiazygos vein

Right greater thoracic splanchnic nerve

Mediastinal pleura

Costal part of parietal pleura

Esophagus

Azygos vein

Thoracic duct

Diaphragmatic part of parietal pleura *(cut away)*

Right leaflet of central tendon

Diaphragmatic part of parietal pleura *(cut away)*

Left leaflet of central tendon

Right phrenic nerve and pericardiacophrenic artery and vein

Mediastinal part of parietal pleura and pericardium *(cut)*

Mediastinal part of parietal pleura and pericardium *(cut)*

Left phrenic nerve and pericardiacophrenic artery and vein

Right costodiaphragmatic recess of pleural cavity

Pericardium

Inferior vena cava (receiving hepatic veins)

Left costomediastinal recess of pleural cavity

Right internal thoracic artery and veins

Transversus thoracis muscle

Right costomediastinal recess of pleural cavity

Left internal thoracic artery and veins

Anterior mediastinum

5th costal cartilage

Sternum

Middle leaflet of central tendon covered by pericardium

Figure 1-15. The thoracic surface of the diaphragm.

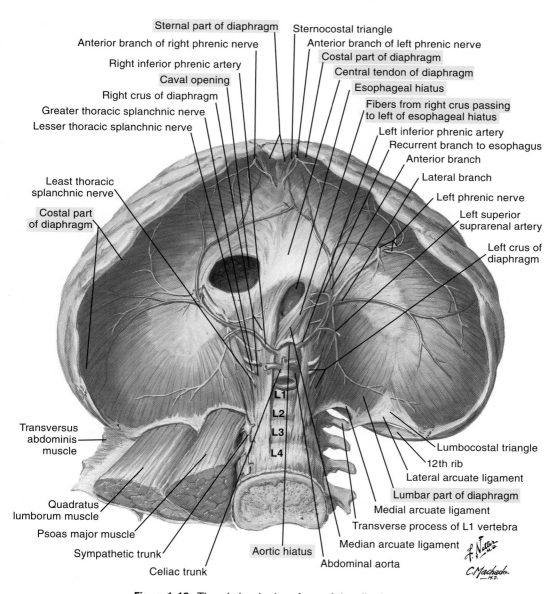

Sternal part of diaphragm
Sternocostal triangle
Anterior branch of right phrenic nerve
Anterior branch of left phrenic nerve
Costal part of diaphragm
Right inferior phrenic artery
Central tendon of diaphragm
Caval opening
Esophageal hiatus
Right crus of diaphragm
Fibers from right crus passing to left of esophageal hiatus
Greater thoracic splanchnic nerve
Lesser thoracic splanchnic nerve
Left inferior phrenic artery
Recurrent branch to esophagus
Anterior branch
Least thoracic splanchnic nerve
Lateral branch
Left phrenic nerve
Costal part of diaphragm
Left superior suprarenal artery
Left crus of diaphragm

Transversus abdominis muscle
Lumbocostal triangle
12th rib
Lateral arcuate ligament
Lumbar part of diaphragm
Quadratus lumborum muscle
Medial arcuate ligament
Transverse process of L1 vertebra
Psoas major muscle
Median arcuate ligament
Sympathetic trunk
Aortic hiatus
Celiac trunk
Abdominal aorta

L1
L2
L3
L4

Figure 1-16. The abdominal surface of the diaphragm.

External Intercostal Muscles (Figures 1-17, 1-18 [p. 54], and 1-19 [p. 55])

Fibers extend from the tubercles of the ribs to the junctions of the costal cartilages and the bony ribs (the costochondral junctions). From there they are replaced by anterior intercostal membranes. A posterior view of the external intercostals reveals that the muscle fibers are oriented inferiorly and laterally (see Figure 1-17, p. 53). Anteriorly, the muscle fibers are oriented inferiorly and medially (see Figure 1-18, p. 54).

There appears to be some regional distribution of the respiratory function of the external and internal intercostals (see next section). The muscle fibers located in more rostral interspaces are inspiratory, and the muscle fibers located in ventral caudal interspaces are expiratory. Inspiratory action raises the rib below; expiratory action lowers the rib above.

The external intercostal muscles are innervated by the intercostal nerves (anterior ramifications of spinal nerves T1 to T11) and the subcostal nerve of T12.

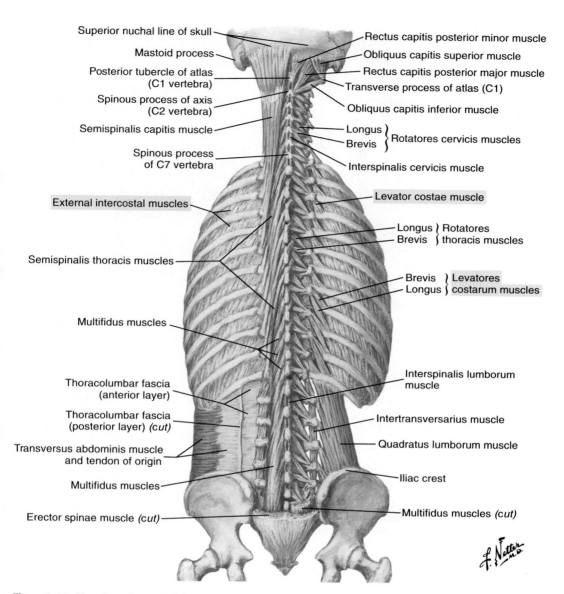

Superior nuchal line of skull

Mastoid process

Posterior tubercle of atlas
(C1 vertebra)

Spinous process of axis
(C2 vertebra)

Semispinalis capitis muscle

Spinous process
of C7 vertebra

External intercostal muscles

Semispinalis thoracis muscles

Multifidus muscles

Thoracolumbar fascia
(anterior layer)

Thoracolumbar fascia
(posterior layer) (cut)

Transversus abdominis muscle
and tendon of origin

Multifidus muscles

Erector spinae muscle (cut)

Rectus capitis posterior minor muscle

Obliquus capitis superior muscle

Rectus capitis posterior major muscle

Transverse process of atlas (C1)

Obliquus capitis inferior muscle

Longus ⎱
Brevis ⎰ Rotatores cervicis muscles

Interspinalis cervicis muscle

Levator costae muscle

Longus ⎱ Rotatores
Brevis ⎰ thoracis muscles

Brevis ⎱ Levatores
Longus ⎰ costarum muscles

Interspinalis lumborum
muscle

Intertransversarius muscle

Quadratus lumborum muscle

Iliac crest

Multifidus muscles (cut)

Figure 1-17. The deep layers of the muscles of the back. Note that posteriorly the muscle fibers of the external intercostals are oriented inferiorly and laterally.

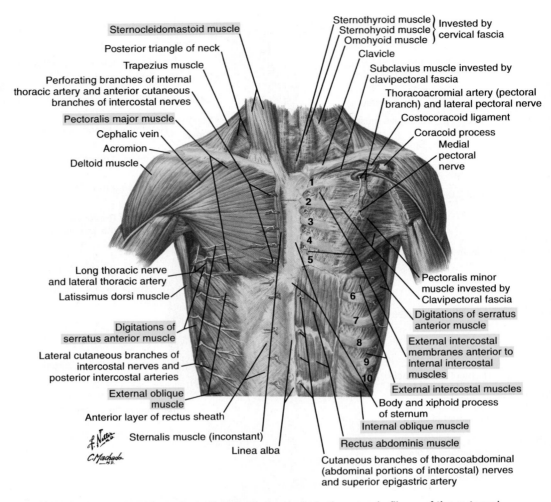

Sternocleidomastoid muscle

Posterior triangle of neck

Trapezius muscle

Perforating branches of internal
thoracic artery and anterior cutaneous
branches of intercostal nerves

Pectoralis major muscle

Cephalic vein

Acromion

Deltoid muscle

Sternothyroid muscle ⎫ Invested by
Sternohyoid muscle ⎬ cervical fascia
Omohyoid muscle ⎭

Clavicle

Subclavius muscle invested by
clavipectoral fascia

Thoracoacromial artery (pectoral
branch) and lateral pectoral nerve

Costocoracoid ligament

Coracoid process
Medial
pectoral
nerve

1
2
3
4
5

Long thoracic nerve
and lateral thoracic artery

Latissimus dorsi muscle

Digitations of
serratus anterior muscle

Lateral cutaneous branches of
intercostal nerves and
posterior intercostal arteries

External oblique
muscle

Anterior layer of rectus sheath

Sternalis muscle (inconstant)

Linea alba

6

7

8

9

10

Pectoralis minor
muscle invested by
Clavipectoral fascia

Digitations of serratus
anterior muscle

External intercostal
membranes anterior to
internal intercostal
muscles

External intercostal muscles

Body and xiphoid process
of sternum

Internal oblique muscle

Rectus abdominis muscle

Cutaneous branches of thoracoabdominal
(abdominal portions of intercostal) nerves
and superior epigastric artery

Figure 1-18. The anterior thoracic wall. Note that anteriorly the muscle fibers of the external
intercostals are oriented inferiorly and medially.

Posterior and Lateral Thoracic Walls

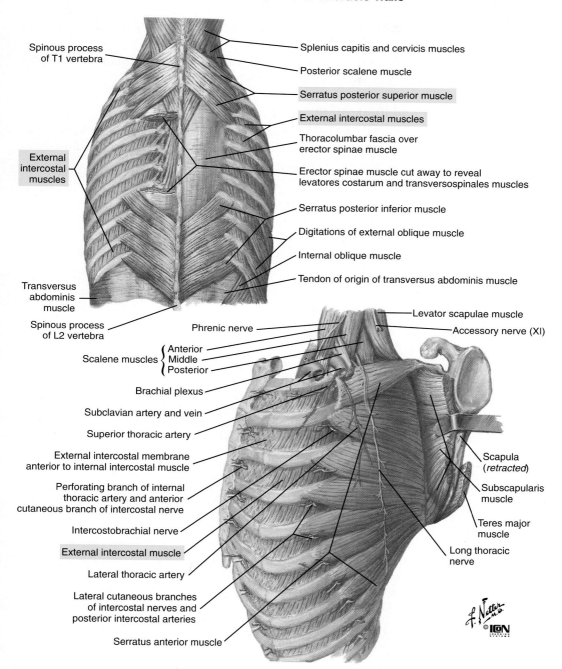

Spinous process of T1 vertebra

External intercostal muscles

Transversus abdominis muscle

Spinous process of L2 vertebra

Splenius capitis and cervicis muscles

Posterior scalene muscle

Serratus posterior superior muscle

External intercostal muscles

Thoracolumbar fascia over erector spinae muscle

Erector spinae muscle cut away to reveal levatores costarum and transversospinales muscles

Serratus posterior inferior muscle

Digitations of external oblique muscle

Internal oblique muscle

Tendon of origin of transversus abdominis muscle

Levator scapulae muscle

Accessory nerve (XI)

Phrenic nerve

Scalene muscles { Anterior / Middle / Posterior

Brachial plexus

Subclavian artery and vein

Superior thoracic artery

External intercostal membrane anterior to internal intercostal muscle

Perforating branch of internal thoracic artery and anterior cutaneous branch of intercostal nerve

Intercostobrachial nerve

External intercostal muscle

Lateral thoracic artery

Lateral cutaneous branches of intercostal nerves and posterior intercostal arteries

Serratus anterior muscle

Scapula (retracted)

Subscapularis muscle

Teres major muscle

Long thoracic nerve

Figure 1-19. The posterior and lateral thoracic walls. Note the external intercostal muscles.

Parasternal (Internal) Intercostal Muscles (Figure 1-20; see also Figure 1-21 [p. 59])

Fibers extend from the costochondral junction and at roughly right angles to the fibers of the internal intercostals (which are absent here) to the sternum; their action is to raise the rib below.

The parasternal intercostal muscles are innervated by the intercostal nerves (anterior ramifications of spinal nerves T1 to T11) and the subcostal nerve of T12.

Accessory Muscles of Inspiration

Accessory muscles of inspiration include a potentially large number of muscles that could have an inspiratory effect on the lungs and thorax. The exact respiratory function, however, of these muscles is not completely understood.

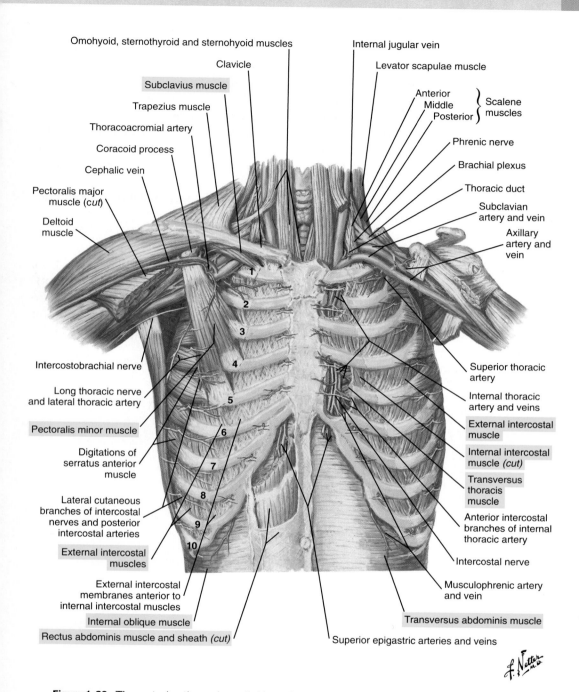

Omohyoid, sternothyroid and sternohyoid muscles

Clavicle

Subclavius muscle

Trapezius muscle

Thoracoacromial artery

Coracoid process

Cephalic vein

Pectoralis major
muscle (*cut*)

Deltoid
muscle

Internal jugular vein

Levator scapulae muscle

Anterior
Middle
Posterior

Scalene
muscles

Phrenic nerve

Brachial plexus

Thoracic duct

Subclavian
artery and vein

Axillary
artery and
vein

Intercostobrachial nerve

Long thoracic nerve
and lateral thoracic artery

Pectoralis minor muscle

Digitations of
serratus anterior
muscle

Lateral cutaneous
branches of intercostal
nerves and posterior
intercostal arteries

External intercostal
muscles

External intercostal
membranes anterior to
internal intercostal muscles

Internal oblique muscle

Rectus abdominis muscle and sheath *(cut)*

Superior thoracic
artery

Internal thoracic
artery and veins

External intercostal
muscle

Internal intercostal
muscle *(cut)*

Transversus
thoracis
muscle

Anterior intercostal
branches of internal
thoracic artery

Intercostal nerve

Musculophrenic artery
and vein

Transversus abdominis muscle

Superior epigastric arteries and veins

Figure 1-20. The anterior thoracic wall. Note the parasternal (internal) intercostal muscles.

Muscles of Expiration

The function of the muscles of expiration is to decrease lung volume.

Internal (Interosseous) Intercostal Muscles (Figure 1-21; see also Figure 1-20, p. 57)

Fibers extend anteriorly (ventrally) from the costochondral junction anteriorly to near the tubercles of the ribs posteriorly (dorsally). Located deep to the external intercostals on the inner surface of the ribs, they travel obliquely and form roughly a right angle to the external intercostals. Interosseous (non-parasternal) internal intercostals have an expiratory function to lower the rib above.

The internal interosseous intercostals are innervated by the intercostal nerves (anterior ramifications of spinal nerves T1 to T11) and the subcostal nerve of T12.

Rectus Abdominis Muscle (see Figure 1-18, p. 54)

The rectus abdominis muscle is formed by large vertical, paired muscles that extend from the pubis to the sternum and the costal cartilages of ribs 5 through 7. These parallel muscles are enclosed in the rectus sheath, which is a continuation of the abdominal aponeurosis of the more laterally located abdominal muscles. The linea alba ("white line") of this sheath separates the right and left muscles. Muscular contraction compresses the abdomen and the rib cage.

The rectus abdominis muscle is innervated by intercostal nerves T7 to T11 and the subcostal nerve of T12.

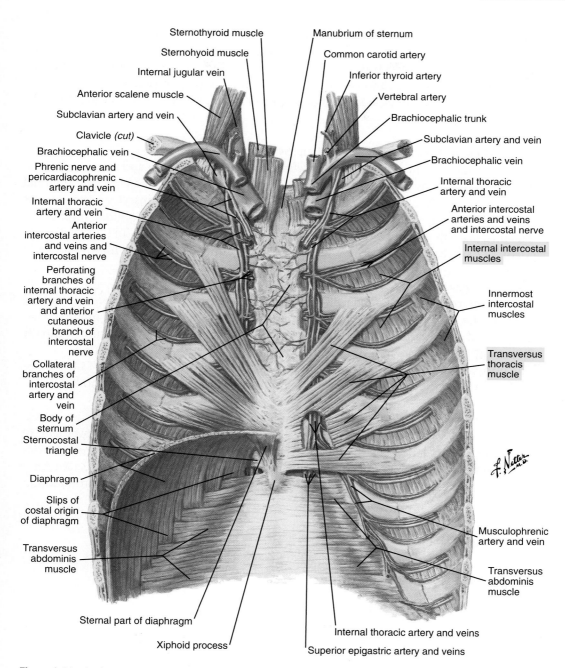

Sternothyroid muscle

Sternohyoid muscle

Internal jugular vein

Anterior scalene muscle

Subclavian artery and vein

Clavicle (cut)

Brachiocephalic vein

Phrenic nerve and pericardiacophrenic artery and vein

Internal thoracic artery and vein

Anterior intercostal arteries and veins and intercostal nerve

Perforating branches of internal thoracic artery and vein and anterior cutaneous branch of intercostal nerve

Collateral branches of intercostal artery and vein

Body of sternum

Sternocostal triangle

Diaphragm

Slips of costal origin of diaphragm

Transversus abdominis muscle

Manubrium of sternum

Common carotid artery

Inferior thyroid artery

Vertebral artery

Brachiocephalic trunk

Subclavian artery and vein

Brachiocephalic vein

Internal thoracic artery and vein

Anterior intercostal arteries and veins and intercostal nerve

Internal intercostal muscles

Innermost intercostal muscles

Transversus thoracis muscle

Musculophrenic artery and vein

Transversus abdominis muscle

Sternal part of diaphragm

Xiphoid process

Internal thoracic artery and veins

Superior epigastric artery and veins

Figure 1-21. An internal view of the anterior thoracic wall. Note the internal (interosseous) intercostal muscles.

External Oblique Muscle (Figures 1-22 and 1-23 [p. 62]; see also Figure 1-18, p. 54)

The external oblique muscle is a large sheetlike muscle that extends from the external surfaces of ribs 5 through 12. It travels obliquely medially and inferiorly to insert on the iliac crest, the inguinal ligament, and the aponeurosis of the external oblique muscle.

The external oblique muscle is innervated by intercostal nerves T7 to T11 and the subcostal nerve of T12.

Internal Oblique Muscle (see Figures 1-18 [p. 54] and 1-23 [p. 62])

The internal oblique muscle is another sheetlike muscle that lies deep and roughly perpendicular to the external oblique muscle. Fibers originate from the iliac crest, the inguinal ligament, and the thoracolumbar fascia (lumbodorsal fascia) and insert on the inferior borders of ribs 10 to 12 and the abdominal aponeurosis of the internal oblique muscle.

The internal oblique muscle is innervated by intercostal nerves T7 to T11 and subcostal nerve of T12 and the iliohypogastric and ilioinguinal branches of the first lumbar nerve.

Transversus Abdominis Muscle (see Figure 1-20, p. 57)

The most internal of the lateral abdominal muscles, the transverse abdominis muscle arises from the thoracolumbar fascia (lumbodorsal fascia), the iliac crest, the inguinal ligament, and the inner surfaces of the cartilages of the lower six ribs to run circumferentially and ventrally to terminate in the aponeurosis of the transversus abdominis muscle.

The transversus abdominis muscle is innervated by intercostal nerves T7 to T11, subcostal nerve of T12, and the iliohypogastric and ilioinguinal branches of the first lumbar nerve.

Tonic abdominal muscle activation, at least in the upright posture, may serve an important "inspiratory" role. Abdominal muscle contraction and the caudal movement of abdominal contents lengthens the diaphragm and increases its force- (pressure) generating capabilities. This "inspiratory" action of abdominal muscles may be important for a variety of respiratory functions, including resting quiet breathing and speech production.

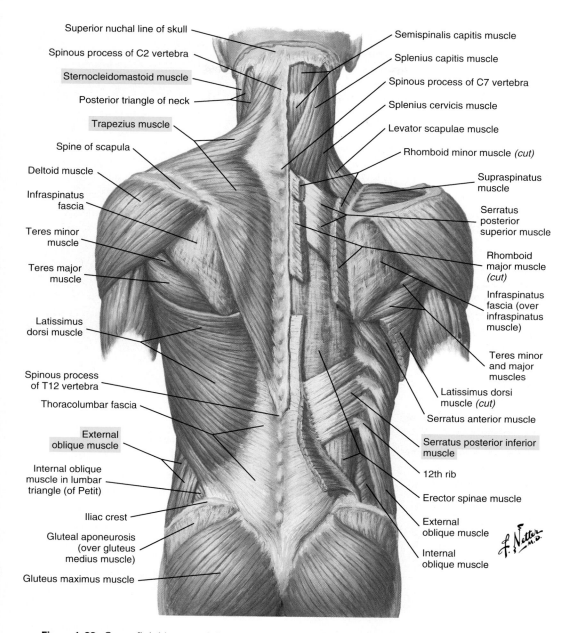

Superior nuchal line of skull

Spinous process of C2 vertebra

Sternocleidomastoid muscle

Posterior triangle of neck

Trapezius muscle

Spine of scapula

Deltoid muscle

Infraspinatus fascia

Teres minor muscle

Teres major muscle

Latissimus dorsi muscle

Spinous process of T12 vertebra

Thoracolumbar fascia

External oblique muscle

Internal oblique muscle in lumbar triangle (of Petit)

Iliac crest

Gluteal aponeurosis (over gluteus medius muscle)

Gluteus maximus muscle

Semispinalis capitis muscle

Splenius capitis muscle

Spinous process of C7 vertebra

Splenius cervicis muscle

Levator scapulae muscle

Rhomboid minor muscle (cut)

Supraspinatus muscle

Serratus posterior superior muscle

Rhomboid major muscle (cut)

Infraspinatus fascia (over infraspinatus muscle)

Teres minor and major muscles

Latissimus dorsi muscle (cut)

Serratus anterior muscle

Serratus posterior inferior muscle

12th rib

Erector spinae muscle

External oblique muscle

Internal oblique muscle

Figure 1-22. Superficial layers of the muscles of the back. Note the external oblique muscle.

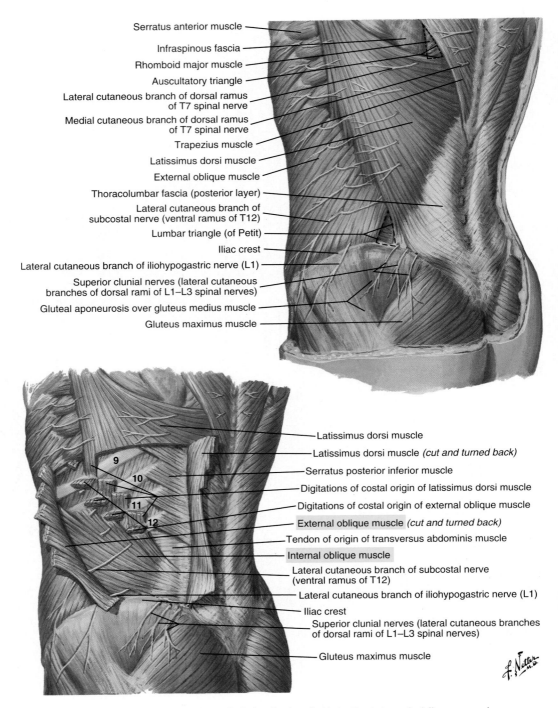

Serratus anterior muscle

Infraspinous fascia

Rhomboid major muscle

Auscultatory triangle

Lateral cutaneous branch of dorsal ramus of T7 spinal nerve

Medial cutaneous branch of dorsal ramus of T7 spinal nerve

Trapezius muscle

Latissimus dorsi muscle

External oblique muscle

Thoracolumbar fascia (posterior layer)

Lateral cutaneous branch of subcostal nerve (ventral ramus of T12)

Lumbar triangle (of Petit)

Iliac crest

Lateral cutaneous branch of iliohypogastric nerve (L1)

Superior clunial nerves (lateral cutaneous branches of dorsal rami of L1–L3 spinal nerves)

Gluteal aponeurosis over gluteus medius muscle

Gluteus maximus muscle

Latissimus dorsi muscle

Latissimus dorsi muscle *(cut and turned back)*

Serratus posterior inferior muscle

Digitations of costal origin of latissimus dorsi muscle

Digitations of costal origin of external oblique muscle

External oblique muscle *(cut and turned back)*

Tendon of origin of transversus abdominis muscle

Internal oblique muscle

Lateral cutaneous branch of subcostal nerve (ventral ramus of T12)

Lateral cutaneous branch of iliohypogastric nerve (L1)

Iliac crest

Superior clunial nerves (lateral cutaneous branches of dorsal rami of L1–L3 spinal nerves)

Gluteus maximus muscle

9
10
11
12

Figure 1-23. The posterolateral abdominal wall. Note the internal oblique muscle.

Primary Muscles of Inspiration (see also Figures 1-26 and 1-27, pp. 68 and 69)

Muscle(s)	Origin	Insertion	Action(s)	Innervation
Diaphragm (see Figures 1-15 [p. 50] and 1-16 [p. 51]) **Three parts** 1. Sternal portion 2. Costal portion 3. Lumbar portion **Central tendon** Aponeurosis in which the three muscular parts insert **Openings** 1. Aortic hiatus 2. Esophageal hiatus 3. Foramen of the inferior vena cava (caval opening)	1. Xiphoid process, inner surface 2. Costal cartilages 3. Adjacent portions of the lower six ribs and superior lumbar vertebrae	All insert into the central tendon	Contraction; pulls central tendon downward, increasing the vertical and anterolateral dimensions of the thorax	Phrenic nerves originating from cervical spinal nerves C3–C5
External intercostals (see Figure 1-20, p. 57)	Inferior surface of the superior rib	Superior surface of the rib below	Expand the rib cage	Intercostal nerves (T1–T11) and subcostal nerve (T12)
Parasternal (internal) intercostals	Inferior surface of rib spaces from the costochondral junction to the sternum	Superior surface of the rib below	Expand the rib cage	Intercostal nerves (T1–T11) and subcostal nerve (T12)

Accessory Muscles of Inspiration

Muscle(s)	Origin	Insertion	Action(s)	Innervation
Pectoralis major (see Figure 1-18, p. 54)	Greater tubercle of the humerus	Clavicle Sternum Cartilages of ribs 1 or 2 through 6 or 7 Aponeurosis of external oblique	With arm fixed, pulls sternum and ribs upward during forced inspiration May also facilitate forced expiration	Lateral and medial pectoral nerves (C5–C8 and T1)
Pectoralis minor (see Figure 1-20, p. 57)	Coracoid process of the scapula	Outer surfaces of ribs 3–5	Elevates ribs 3–5	Lateral and medial pectoral nerves (C5–C8 and T1)
Levator costae (levatores costarum) (see Figure 1-17, p. 53)	C7, T1–T11 vertebrae	Laterally to the dorsal surface of the rib below	Elevates the ribs	Intercostal nerves (T2–T12)
Serratus posterior superior (Figure 1-24; see also Figure 1-20, p. 57)	By aponeurosis from vertebrae C6–T2	Downward and laterally to superior border of ribs 2–5, near costal angle	Elevates ribs to which it attaches	Intercostal nerves (T2–T5)
Serratus anterior (see Figure 1-18, p. 54)	Inner, medial border of the scapula	Eight or nine upper ribs	Elevates upper ribs	Long thoracic nerve (C5–C7)
Subclavius (see Figure 1-20, p. 57)	Small muscle from inferior surface of the clavicle	First rib at costochondral junction	Elevates first rib	Subclavian nerve (C5–C6)
Sternocleidomastoid (Figure 1-25, p. 66; see also Figure 1-18, p. 54)	Mastoid process of temporal bone	Sternum and clavicle	Raises the sternum and thus the ribs	Spinal accessory nerve (cranial nerve XI) and cervical spinal nerves C2–C4
Trapezius (see Figure 1-22, p. 61)	External occipital protuberance and superior nuchal line of the occipital bone Spinous processes of C7–T12 vertebrae	Lateral one-third of the clavicle Acromion and spine of the scapula	Tilts the head backward and laterally Rotates the scapula Elevates and depresses the shoulders Maintains trunk stability for respiration	Spinal accessory nerve (XI)
Scalene muscles*: anterior, middle, and posterior (see Figure 1-25, p. 66)	Transverse processes of cervical vertebrae C2–C7	Upper surfaces of first and second ribs	Elevate the ribs	Anterior: cervical spinal nerves C4–C6 Middle: C3–C8 Posterior: C6–C8

*Often listed as accessory muscles of respiration, scalene muscles have been shown to be consistently active during resting inspiration in a variety of animal species, including humans. Some authors therefore consider them to be primary muscles of inspiration.

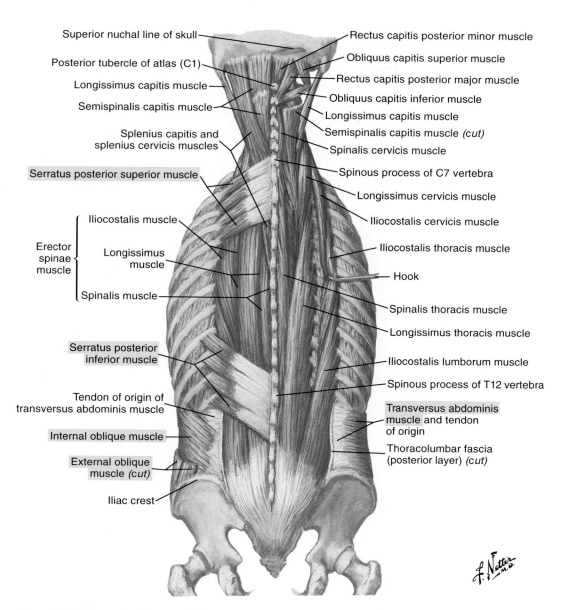

Superior nuchal line of skull

Posterior tubercle of atlas (C1)

Longissimus capitis muscle

Semispinalis capitis muscle

Splenius capitis and splenius cervicis muscles

Serratus posterior superior muscle

Erector spinae muscle {
Iliocostalis muscle

Longissimus muscle

Spinalis muscle
}

Serratus posterior inferior muscle

Tendon of origin of transversus abdominis muscle

Internal oblique muscle

External oblique muscle *(cut)*

Iliac crest

Rectus capitis posterior minor muscle

Obliquus capitis superior muscle

Rectus capitis posterior major muscle

Obliquus capitis inferior muscle

Longissimus capitis muscle

Semispinalis capitis muscle *(cut)*

Spinalis cervicis muscle

Spinous process of C7 vertebra

Longissimus cervicis muscle

Iliocostalis cervicis muscle

Iliocostalis thoracis muscle

Hook

Spinalis thoracis muscle

Longissimus thoracis muscle

Iliocostalis lumborum muscle

Spinous process of T12 vertebra

Transversus abdominis muscle and tendon of origin

Thoracolumbar fascia (posterior layer) *(cut)*

Figure 1-24. Intermediate layers of the muscles of the back. Note the serratus posterior superior muscle.

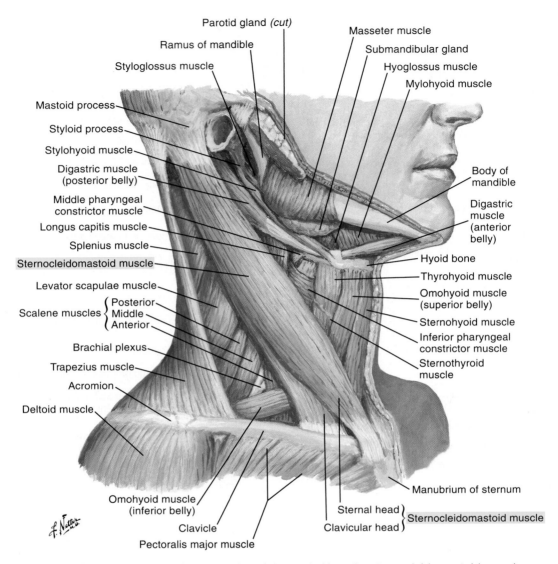

Parotid gland *(cut)*

Ramus of mandible

Styloglossus muscle

Masseter muscle

Submandibular gland

Hyoglossus muscle

Mylohyoid muscle

Mastoid process

Styloid process

Stylohyoid muscle

Digastric muscle
(posterior belly)

Middle pharyngeal
constrictor muscle

Longus capitis muscle

Splenius muscle

Sternocleidomastoid muscle

Levator scapulae muscle

Scalene muscles { Posterior
Middle
Anterior

Brachial plexus

Trapezius muscle

Acromion

Deltoid muscle

Body of
mandible

Digastric
muscle
(anterior
belly)

Hyoid bone

Thyrohyoid muscle

Omohyoid muscle
(superior belly)

Sternohyoid muscle

Inferior pharyngeal
constrictor muscle

Sternothyroid
muscle

Omohyoid muscle
(inferior belly)

Clavicle

Pectoralis major muscle

Sternal head }
Clavicular head } Sternocleidomastoid muscle

Manubrium of sternum

Figure 1-25. A lateral view of the muscles of the neck. Note the sternocleidomastoid muscle.

Muscles of Expiration

Muscle(s)	Origin	Insertion	Action(s)	Innervation
Internal (interosseous) intercostals (see Figure 1-21, p. 59)	Inner superior surface of the rib below	Inner inferior surface of the rib above	Pull ribs downward, fixes ribs	Intercostal nerves (T1–T11) Subcostal nerve (T12)
Rectus abdominis (Figures 1-26 [p. 68] and 1-27 [p. 69]; see also Figure 1-18, p. 54)	Pubic symphysis and pubic crest	Costal cartilages or ribs 5–7 and xiphoid process of the sternum	Compresses abdomen and rib cage	Intercostal nerves (T7–T11) Subcostal nerve (T12)
External oblique (see Figures 1-18 [p. 54], 1-26 [p. 68], and 1-27 [p. 69])	External surfaces of the eight lowest ribs	Iliac crest Inguinal ligament Aponeurosis of the external oblique	Compresses abdomen and rib cage	Intercostal nerves (T7–T11) Subcostal nerve (T12)
Internal oblique (see Figures 1-18 [p. 54], 1-26 [p. 68], and 1-27 [p. 69])	Iliac crest Inguinal ligaments Thoracolumbar fascia	Costal cartilages of the lowest three or four ribs	Brings costal cartilages closer to the pubis Compresses abdomen	Intercostal nerves (T7–T11) Subcostal nerve (T12) First lumbar spinal nerve, L1 (iliohypogastric and ilioinguinal branches)
Transversus abdominis (see Figures 1-18 [p. 54], 1-26 [p. 68], and 1-27 [p. 69])	Iliac crest Inguinal ligaments Thoracolumbar fascia Cartilages of the lower six ribs	Aponeurosis of the transversus abdominis	Compresses the abdomen and rib cage	Intercostal nerves (T7–T11) Subcostal nerve (T12) First lumbar spinal nerve, L1 (iliohypogastric and ilioinguinal branches)
Transverse thoracis (triangularis sterni) (see Figure 1-21, p. 59)	Internal surface of the rib cage from the sternum and costal cartilages 5–7	Internal surface of costal cartilages and adjacent portions of ribs 2–6	Compresses rib cage	Intercostal nerves (T2–T6)
Serratus posterior inferior (see Figure 1-22, p. 61)	By aponeurosis from vertebrae T11–L2/3	Superiorly and laterally to the inferior surface of the lowest 3 to 4 ribs	Lowers ribs	Intercostal nerves (T9–T11) and subcostal nerve (T12)

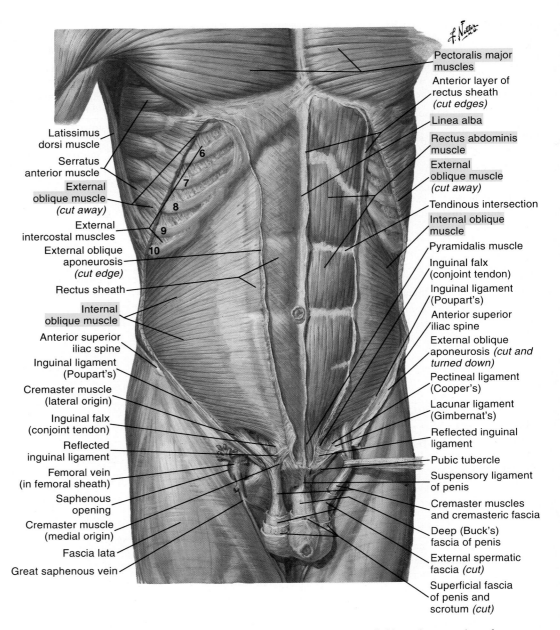

Pectoralis major muscles

Anterior layer of rectus sheath (cut edges)

Linea alba

Rectus abdominis muscle

External oblique muscle (cut away)

Tendinous intersection

Internal oblique muscle

Pyramidalis muscle

Inguinal falx (conjoint tendon)

Inguinal ligament (Poupart's)

Anterior superior iliac spine

External oblique aponeurosis (cut and turned down)

Pectineal ligament (Cooper's)

Lacunar ligament (Gimbernat's)

Reflected inguinal ligament

Pubic tubercle

Suspensory ligament of penis

Cremaster muscles and cremasteric fascia

Deep (Buck's) fascia of penis

External spermatic fascia (cut)

Superficial fascia of penis and scrotum (cut)

Latissimus dorsi muscle

Serratus anterior muscle

External oblique muscle (cut away)

External intercostal muscles

External oblique aponeurosis (cut edge)

Rectus sheath

Internal oblique muscle

Anterior superior iliac spine

Inguinal ligament (Poupart's)

Cremaster muscle (lateral origin)

Inguinal falx (conjoint tendon)

Reflected inguinal ligament

Femoral vein (in femoral sheath)

Saphenous opening

Cremaster muscle (medial origin)

Fascia lata

Great saphenous vein

6
7
8
9
10

Figure 1-26. An intermediate dissection of the anterior abdominal wall. Note the muscles of expiration.

Section above arcuate line

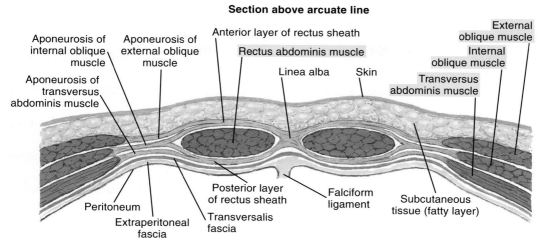

Aponeurosis of internal oblique muscle splits to form anterior and posterior layers of rectus sheath. Aponeurosis of external oblique muscle joins anterior layer of sheath; aponeurosis of transversus abdominis muscle joins posterior layer. Anterior and posterior layers of rectus sheath unite medially to form linea alba.

Section below arcuate line

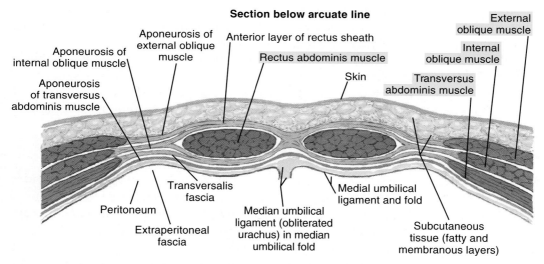

Aponeurosis of internal oblique muscle does not split at this level but passes completely anterior to rectus abdominis muscle and is fused there with both aponeurosis of external oblique muscle and that of transversus abdominis muscle. Thus, posterior wall of rectus sheath is absent below arcuate line, and rectus abdominis muscle lies on transversalis fascia.

Figure 1-27. Cross-sections of the rectus sheath. Note the aponeurosis of the external oblique muscle.

■ RESPIRATORY VOLUMES AND CAPACITIES

Volumes (Figure 1-28)

The different respiratory volumes are mutually exclusive, meaning that they do not overlap, and are as follows:
- **Tidal** volume is the volume (or amount) of air inspired or expired during normal, quiet breathing.
- **Inspiratory reserve** volume is the maximum amount of air that can be inspired above normal inspiratory tidal volume.
- **Expiratory reserve** volume is the maximum amount of air that can be expired below normal expiratory tidal volume.
- **Residual** volume is the amount of air remaining in the lungs after a maximal forced expiration (thus the lungs cannot be completely emptied voluntarily).

Capacities

Respiratory capacities are sums of volumes and are measured during the following pulmonary function tests:
- **Inspiratory** capacity is the total amount of air that can be inspired after a tidal expiration (tidal volume + inspiratory reserve volume).
- **Functional residual** capacity is the amount of air remaining in the lungs after a normal tidal expiration (expiratory reserve volume + residual volume).
- **Vital** capacity is the total amount of air that can be forcibly expired after a maximal inspiration (inspiratory reserve volume + tidal volume + expiratory reserve volume).
- **Total lung** capacity is the total amount of air after a maximal inspiration. It is the sum of all volumes (residual volume + expiratory reserve volume + tidal volume + inspiratory reserve volume).

Other Functional Measures

Minute ventilation is the amount of air moved into or out of the lungs per minute and is calculated by multiplying tidal volume by breaths per minute (respiratory rate).

Physiological dead space is the volume of air remaining in the conducting airways (such as the bronchi, trachea, pharynx, and so on) that does not reach the alveoli and participate in gas exchange (referred to as *anatomical dead space*) and the volume of air that reaches the alveoli but does not exchange carbon dioxide or oxygen (referred to as *alveolar dead space*). Physiological dead space is roughly equal to anatomical dead space in healthy individuals.

Alveolar ventilation is the volume of air per minute that reaches the alveoli *and* takes part in gas exchange. It is calculated by subtracting physiological dead space volume from tidal volume and multiplying by respiratory rate.

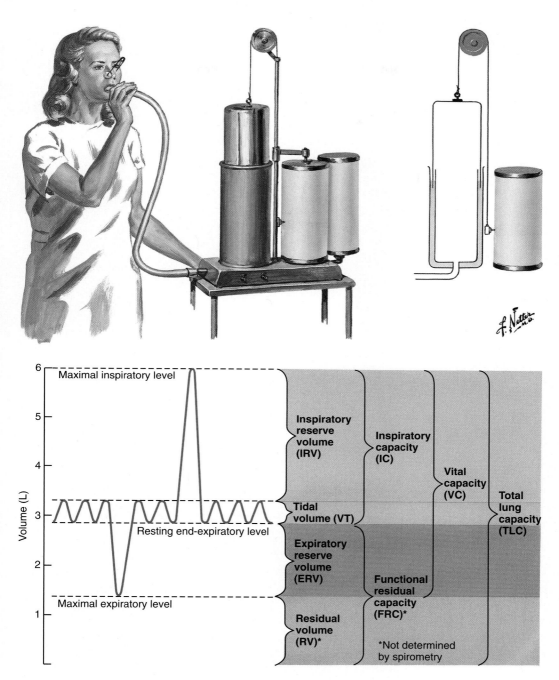

Figure 1-28. Spirometry: lung volumes and subdivisions.

PHONATORY SYSTEM

2

■ OVERVIEW

The larynx has three primary biological functions. First, it prevents foreign objects from entering the airway (e.g., during swallowing). Second, it traps air in the lungs and stabilizes the torso for physical exertion, such as lifting heavy objects, and third, it modifies upper airway resistance during the inspiratory and expiratory phases of breathing to ensure adequate gas exchange.

Superimposed on these more primitive functions is the use of the vocal folds for sound generation. To produce voiced sounds, the vocal folds are closed (adducted), and subglottal pressure (the pressure buildup beneath the folds) overcomes the resistance of the folds, and they open, which releases a burst of compressed air into the supraglottal space known as the *vocal tract*. The elastic recoil of the stretched tissue combined with Bernoulli forces returns the folds to their closed position. The cycle then repeats itself when subglottal pressure overcomes the resistance of the continuously adducted vocal folds. Driven by these pressure pulses, the air above the vocal folds vibrates and provides the acoustic sound source. The sound generated by the vibrating vocal folds is a complex sound that contains a fundamental frequency and harmonics with significant energy up to approximately 4500 Hz. It is this complex acoustical signal that is modified by the resonant characteristics of the vocal tract to produce specific sounds such as vowels.

Variations in fundamental frequency (the rate of opening and closing of the vibrating vocal folds) and its perceptual correlate pitch serve important signaling roles in speech production. Changes in fundamental frequency result from changes in the length and tension of the vocal folds, which in turn results from a complex interplay between intrinsic and extrinsic laryngeal muscles, with the cricothyroid and thyroarytenoid playing crucial roles. Changes in subglottal pressure also influence fundamental frequency.

Increases in vocal intensity (loudness) are related to increased expiratory drive and greater medial compression and tension of the adducted vocal folds. Increased subglottal pressure creates greater lateral excursion of vocal folds during opening and, consequently, larger pressure pulses (and associated acoustic energy) entering the supralaryngeal vocal tract.

The anatomical terms *abduction* and *adduction* refer to midline movements of the vocal folds to open and closed positions, respectively, by muscular forces. During phonation, the vocal folds are brought to a position of adduction and they remain in this state during vocal fold vibration. The opening and closing of the vocal folds superimposed on the adduction of the vocal folds occurs through the complex interaction of the mechanical and aerodynamic factors described previously.

It should be noted that the laryngeal system also functions as an articulator, rapidly adducting and abducting the vocal folds for voiced (those that involve vocal fold vibration) and unvoiced sounds, respectively, during connected speech. This activity must be precisely timed with respiratory drive and supralaryngeal articulatory movements for specific sound production. The vocal folds also serve a vital function for swallowing. They protect the airway against the penetration and aspiration of foods and liquids.

The components of the phonatory system are presented in this section, including the structural framework of the larynx, the vocal folds, and the associated laryngeal muscles.

■ LARYNX (Figure 2-1; see also Figure 2-2, p. 79)

The larynx is approximately 5 cm in length and extends from the level of the third or fourth cervical vertebra to the sixth. It is located in the anterior portion of the neck, in front of the pharynx, above the trachea, and below the hyoid bone. The larynx functions as a two-way valve for the respiratory airway. It can function in this way because of two mobile muscular (and other soft tissue) bands called the *vocal folds*.

The structural framework of the larynx is composed of several paired and unpaired laryngeal cartilages and associated membranes and ligaments, as follows:
- Larger unpaired cartilages (major structure):
  - Thyroid cartilage
  - Cricoid cartilages
  - Epiglottis
- Smaller paired cartilages:
  - Arytenoid cartilages
  - Corniculate, or Santorini's, cartilages
  - Cuneiform cartilages
  - Triticeal cartilages

The epiglottis and the corniculate, cuneiform, and triticeal cartilages are formed of elastic cartilage; the rest are formed of hyaline cartilage, which may calcify with advancing age, with the exception of the arytenoid cartilages, which have a dense concentration of elastic cartilage in their vocal processes.

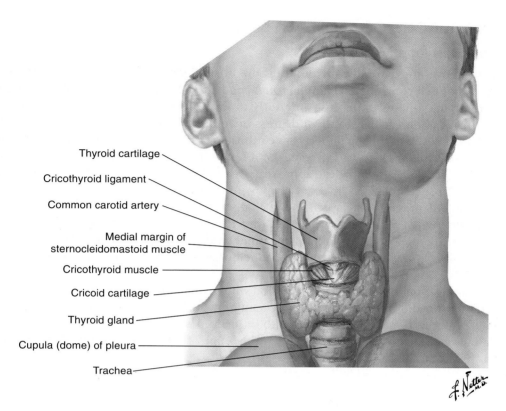

Thyroid cartilage

Cricothyroid ligament

Common carotid artery

Medial margin of
sternocleidomastoid muscle

Cricothyroid muscle

Cricoid cartilage

Thyroid gland

Cupula (dome) of pleura

Trachea

Figure 2-1. Position of the larynx, anterior view, in situ.

■ CARTILAGES OF THE LARYNX (Figure 2-2)

Thyroid Cartilage

Situated above and partially surrounding the cricoid cartilage, the thyroid cartilage is composed of two convex lateral lamina roughly quadrilateral in shape: the quadrilateral or thyroid lamina. These lamina fuse anteriorly to form the thyroid angle of approximately 120 degrees in adult females and 90 degrees in adult males. The more acute angle in the male (which develops during puberty) as contrasted to the female reflects longer and more massive vocal folds. This in turn relates to a lower fundamental frequency of vocal fold vibration (pitch) in adult males (approximately 125 Hz) versus females (approximately 210 Hz) because frequency is inversely proportional to mass.

- A palpable depression or "notch" on the superior surface of the two fused lamina is called the *thyroid notch*. This notch lies directly superior to the laryngeal prominence, or "Adam's apple," which is more prominent (and visible) in males versus females. The notch is at the approximate level of the horizontally oriented vocal folds (see later section).
- There are two pairs of horns: two superior, which articulate with the hyoid bone via the lateral thyrohyoid ligament (lateral thickening of the thyrohyoid membrane), and two smaller inferior horns that articulate with the cricoid cartilage.
- The oblique line on the lateral surface is the point of attachment of the sternothyroid, thyrohyoid, and thyropharyngeus muscles.
- The anterior cricothyroid ligament attaches the thyroid with the cricoid anteriorly.

Cricoid Cartilage

Cricoid cartilage is situated just above the superior tracheal cartilage. It forms the inferior portion of the larynx and attaches to the trachea via the cricotracheal membrane or ligament. Cricoid cartilage forms a complete "signet" ring, as follows:

- The front is composed of a low anterior arch.
- The back is composed of a taller posterior quadrate (cricoid) lamina.
  The two paired points of articulation with synovial joints are as follows:
- One point for the arytenoid cartilages is located on the superior surface of the quadrate lamina and allows for adduction and abduction of the paired vocal folds.
- One point for the inferior horns of the thyroid cartilage is located on the lateral surface and allows for movement between the cricoid and thyroid cartilages to adjust the length and tension of the vocal folds.

Arytenoid Cartilages

The arytenoid cartilages are small pyramidal cartilages with the inferior concave surface or base resting on the convex arytenoid facets on the lateral border of the superior surface of the posterior quadrate lamina of the cricoid. The location and movement of these two cartilages are crucial to laryngeal function.

Three processes of the arytenoid cartilages are as follows:
1. The apex (the pyramid's summit) is the superior process.
2. The muscular process (site of muscular insertion) extends laterally.
3. The vocal process (site of vocal fold insertion) extends anteriorly.

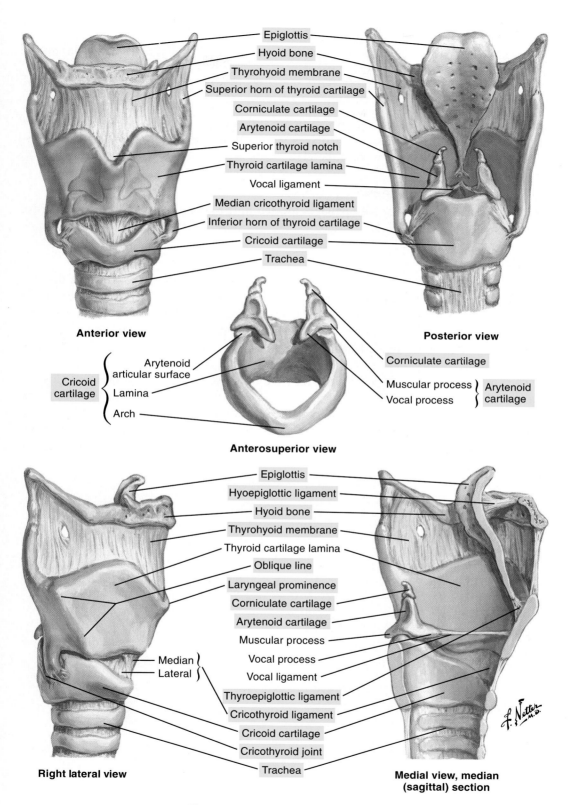

Anterior view

Posterior view

Epiglottis
Hyoid bone
Thyrohyoid membrane
Superior horn of thyroid cartilage
Corniculate cartilage
Arytenoid cartilage
Superior thyroid notch
Thyroid cartilage lamina
Vocal ligament
Median cricothyroid ligament
Inferior horn of thyroid cartilage
Cricoid cartilage
Trachea

Cricoid cartilage
Arytenoid articular surface
Lamina
Arch

Corniculate cartilage
Muscular process
Vocal process
Arytenoid cartilage

Anterosuperior view

Right lateral view

Medial view, median (sagittal) section

Epiglottis
Hyoepiglottic ligament
Hyoid bone
Thyrohyoid membrane
Thyroid cartilage lamina
Oblique line
Laryngeal prominence
Corniculate cartilage
Arytenoid cartilage
Muscular process
Vocal process
Median
Lateral
Vocal ligament
Thyroepiglottic ligament
Cricothyroid ligament
Cricoid cartilage
Cricothyroid joint
Trachea

Figure 2-2. The laryngeal cartilages.

Legends and labels of certain figures are highlighted in yellow to emphasize the related elements in the corresponding text.

Corniculate, or Santorini's, Cartilages

Corniculate cartilages, or Santorini's cartilages, are elastic conical-shaped cartilages on the apex of the arytenoid cartilages.

Cuneiform Cartilages

Cuneiform cartilages are covered in soft tissue and situated within the aryepiglottic folds anterosuperior to the corniculate cartilages. They cannot be directly seen, but their presence is indicated by the cuneiform tubercles.

Triticeal (Tritiate) Cartilages

The triticeal cartilages are small cartilages located in the lateral hyothyroid ligaments (not present in all people).

Epiglottis

The epiglottis is a flexible elastic cartilage situated behind the median portion of the thyroid cartilage, which it exceeds superiorly. It is attached to the inner medial surface of the thyroid angle by the thyroepiglottic ligament. The epiglottis extends obliquely superiorly and posteriorly and attaches to the hyoid bone via the hyoepiglottic ligament. The aryepiglottic fold extends from the lateral margins of the epiglottis to the apexes of the arytenoids.

The epiglottis is attached to the root of the tongue via the median and lateral glossoepiglottic folds to create the valleculae (see Part 3: Articulatory System, pp. 105–167). The pyriform (piriform) sinus (fossa) is a small lateral recess between the aryepiglottic fold (medially) and the thyroid cartilage and thyrohyoid membrane (laterally). The "tipping" of the epiglottis during laryngeal elevation for swallowing may assist in protecting the upper airway.

■ HYOID BONE (see Figure 2-2, p. 79)

The hyoid bone provides support for the tongue and the larynx, but it is not generally considered as a part of the larynx. It is a "floating" bone that does not have direct contact with any other bone. It is instead attached by a complex system of muscles and ligaments from the tongue and the extrinsic muscles of larynx and other facial, cranial, and skeletal structures. It is therefore a very mobile structure acted on by several muscle systems.

Located in the neck at the level of the third cervical vertebrae, it is oriented horizontally and has a horseshoe-like shape with the following components:

- A rectangular body (corpus)
- A pair of lesser horns (cornu)
- A pair of greater horns (cornu)

An additional description of the hyoid bone is provided in Part 3: Articulatory System, pp. 105–167.

■ TYPES OF JOINTS (see Figure 2-2, p. 79)

Three types of joints exist, each differing in its degree of mobility, as follows:
1. Fibrous joint is immobile.
2. Cartilaginous joint is slightly mobile.
3. Synovial joint is highly mobile.

The two important points of articulation and associated joints of the larynx are as follows:

- **Cricothyroid** is the synovial joint between the lesser thyroid horn (inferior horn) of the thyroid cartilage and the articular facets of the cricoid. This joint allows for two types of movements: (1) forward "bending" of the thyroid over the cricoid and (2) anteroposterior gliding of the thyroid in the horizontal axis. Each of these movements potentially impacts the length (and tension) of the vocal folds.
- **Cricoarytenoid** is the synovial joint between the base of the arytenoids and the superior surface of the quadrate lamina of the cricoid. It allows rocking toward (inferiorly medially) or away from (superiorly laterally) the interior of the cricoid, bringing the vocal processes and, consequently, the vocal folds into adduction and abduction, respectively.

■ LIGAMENTS AND MEMBRANES (see Figure 2-2, p. 79)

The laryngeal cartilages are linked together and to adjacent structures by extrinsic and intrinsic ligaments and membranes.

Extrinsic Ligaments and Membranes

The function of the extrinsic ligaments and membranes is to suspend and link the larynx to the following adjacent structures.

Thyrohyoid (Hyothyroid) Ligament

The thyrohyoid membrane lies between the superior border of the thyroid cartilage and the hyoid bone. It becomes thicker medially to form the median (middle) thyrohyoid ligament. This membrane also becomes thicker posteriorly and laterally to form the lateral thyrohyoid ligaments, which link the superior horn of the thyroid to the hyoid bone.

Hyoepiglottic Ligament

The hyoepiglottic ligament links the anterior surface of the epiglottis to the inner surface of the superior surface of the body of the hyoid.

Cricotracheal Membrane

The cricotracheal membrane joins the superior border of the first tracheal ring to the inferior surface of the cricoid.

Intrinsic Ligaments and Membranes

The function of the intrinsic ligaments and membranes is to link and support the laryngeal cartilages. Most of the intrinsic laryngeal membranes arise from a sheet of connective tissue called the *elastic membrane.* Its inferior division is called the *conus elasticus,* and the superior portion is called the *quadrangular membrane.*

Quadrangular Membrane

The quadrangular membrane is formed of paired membranes from the lateral edge of the epiglottis and angle of the thyroid cartilage. These extend posteriorly and inferiorly to the corniculate cartilages and the medial borders of the arytenoids. The quadrangular membrane is wider superiorly and narrows inferiorly to form the ventricular, or false, vocal folds.

The aryepiglottic folds form the free superior border of the quadrangular membrane and extend from the lateral surface of the epiglottis to the apexes of the arytenoids. The cuneiform cartilages are embedded in these folds.

Conus Elasticus, Cricovocal, or Lateral Cricothyroid Ligament or Membrane

The conus elasticus is a cone-shaped, thin continuous membrane that extends from the superior surface of the cricoid cartilage, terminating medially as the vocal ligaments. These ligaments extend from the vocal process of the arytenoid cartilages to the angle of the thyroid cartilage and form a portion of the vocal folds.

The conus elasticus is sometimes considered to include the anterior or medial cricothyroid ligament (see Figure 2-2, p. 79 and Figure 2-6, p. 93), which is a well-defined elastic tissue that extends from the superior surface of the cricoid arch to the inferior border of the thyroid cartilage near the angle of the thyroid.

■ VOCAL FOLDS (Figures 2-3, 2-4 [p. 86], and 2-5 [p. 87]; see also Figure 2-6 [p. 93])

Throughout this atlas, the term *vocal folds* is used to designate the structures involved in the generation of the laryngeal sound source of speech. Although the term *vocal cords* is perhaps better known, the term *vocal folds* is the more appropriate anatomical term to designate these key laryngeal structures.

The use of the term *vocal cords* may have come from the early visual inspections of the larynx and the appearance of the thickened vocal ligaments, which resemble "cords." Since then, our understanding of the structure and function of the vibration of the vocal folds has advanced, and we now know that these are complex structures in the form of folds composed of muscles, ligaments, and membranes.

The larynx serves several primary biological functions, including protecting the airway. Simple cords obviously cannot prevent the entry of foreign objects into the lower airway, but vocal folds forming a laryngeal valve can. There are actually two pairs of vocal folds arranged in parallel and in an anteroposterior orientation, which can be most clearly seen in a coronal section of the larynx (see Figure 2-5, p. 87) and described as the following:

- The false vocal folds (or ventricular folds) do not normally generate a sound source.
- The true vocal folds are inferior to the false vocal folds and are separated from the ventricular folds by a small fissure called the *ventricle.*
- The supraglottic region is superior to the ventricle.
- The quadrangular membrane is located above the vocal folds.
- The aryepiglottic folds form the "collar" or point of constriction to the entryway to the larynx.
- The subglottic region extends from the inferior border of the true folds to the inferior border of the cricoid cartilage.
- The conus elasticus is the membranous covering in the subglottic region.
- The glottic region corresponds to the space between the true vocal folds, which is also known as the *glottis.*

Although estimates vary, vocal fold lengths generally range from:

- Men: 17 to 25 mm
- Women: 13 to 18 mm

The thickness of the vocal folds is approximately 5 mm.

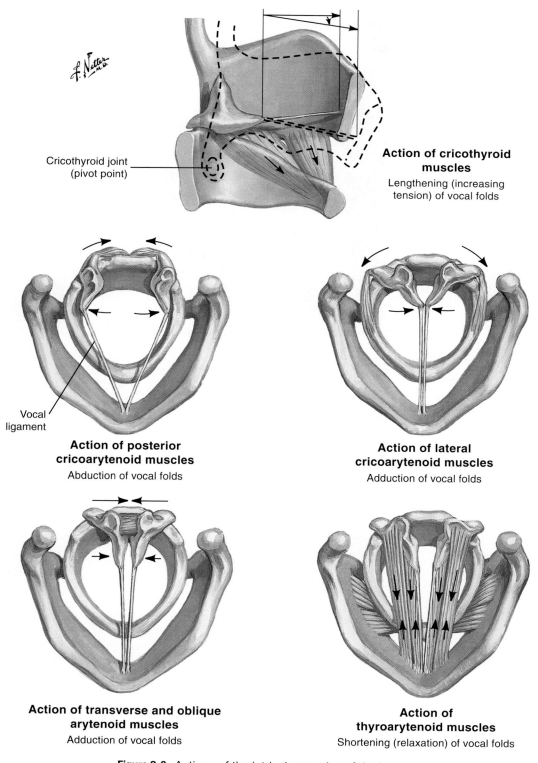

Cricothyroid joint
(pivot point)

**Action of cricothyroid
muscles**
Lengthening (increasing
tension) of vocal folds

Vocal
ligament

**Action of posterior
cricoarytenoid muscles**
Abduction of vocal folds

**Action of lateral
cricoarytenoid muscles**
Adduction of vocal folds

**Action of transverse and oblique
arytenoid muscles**
Adduction of vocal folds

**Action of
thyroarytenoid muscles**
Shortening (relaxation) of vocal folds

Figure 2-3. Actions of the intrinsic muscles of the larynx.

Laryngoscopic View of the Larynx: Inspiration

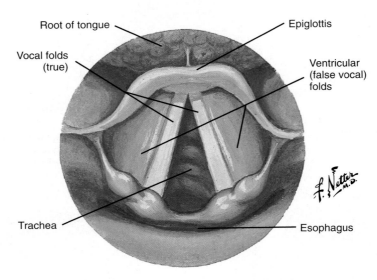

Root of tongue

Epiglottis

Vocal folds (true)

Ventricular (false vocal) folds

Trachea

Esophagus

Figure 2-4. Abduction of the vocal folds during inspiration.

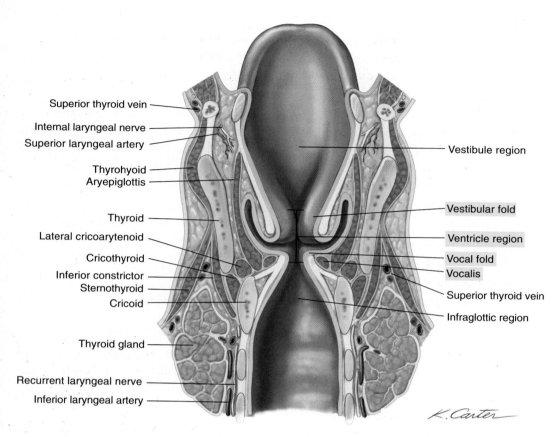

Superior thyroid vein
Internal laryngeal nerve
Superior laryngeal artery
Thyrohyoid
Aryepiglottis
Thyroid
Lateral cricoarytenoid
Cricothyroid
Inferior constrictor
Sternothyroid
Cricoid
Thyroid gland
Recurrent laryngeal nerve
Inferior laryngeal artery

Vestibule region
Vestibular fold
Ventricle region
Vocal fold
Vocalis
Superior thyroid vein
Infraglottic region

K. Carter

Figure 2-5. The coronal section of the larynx. Note the vestibular and true vocal folds.

Tissue Layers of the Vocal Folds

The vocal folds of an adult are composed of five layers of tissue: (1) the epithelium; (2) the superficial layer; (3) the intermediate layer; (4) the deep layer; and (5) the thyroarytenoid, or vocalis, muscle. Each layer differs in terms of thickness and rigidity.

Epithelium

The epithelium is stratified, has a thickness of approximately 0.05 to 0.10 mm, and is the rigid layer that maintains the shape of the vocal folds. Under the epithelium is a composite structure of three layers called the *lamina propria.* The lamina propria has a thickness of 1 mm. The epithelium is attached to the superficial layer of the lamina propria by a complex basement membrane.

Superficial Layer (Reinke's Space)

The superficial layer, or Reinke's space, is composed of loosely organized cells that form a gelatinous-like matrix approximately 0.5 mm thick. This layer is responsible for much of the vibratory movements of the vocal folds.

Intermediate Layer

The intermediate layer is formed by elastic fibers and in cross-section appears to resemble a bunch of cut, supple rubber bands.

Deep Layer

The deep layer is formed primarily by collagen fibers, with the consistency of a group of large cotton threads. The intermediate and deep layers form the vocal ligament and together are approximately 1 to 2 mm thick.

Thyroarytenoid, or Vocalis, Muscle

The thyroarytenoid, or vocalis, muscle is located under the vocal ligament. Muscular fibers form the bulk of the vocal folds and have the consistency of a packet of rigid rubber bands.

A variety of biomechanical models have been proposed to explain the vibratory or oscillatory behavior of the vocal folds during phonation. Within a biomechanical perspective, the vocal folds can be grouped into the following functional divisions:

- The **cover,** surface, or mucosa consists of epithelium and superficial layer of lamina propria (layers 1 and 2).
- The **transition** or vocal ligament consists of intermediate and deep layers of lamina propria (layers 3 and 4).
- The **body** or muscle consists of the thyroarytenoid muscle (layer 5).

Another two-layer biomechanical scheme combines layers 1 through 3 to form the **cover** and layers 4 and 5 to form the **body.**

From a simplified biomechanical perspective, changes in the length, stiffness (tension), and mass of the vocal folds determine the fundamental frequency of vocal fold vibration and its perceptual correlate of pitch. These parameters, and thus fundamental frequency, are thought to be regulated primarily through activation of the cricothyroid and thyroarytenoid muscles, with the cricothyroid muscle being the primary controller.

The cricothyroid muscle controls fundamental frequency by lengthening and thinning the vocal folds, which increases longitudinal tension and results in increased fundamental frequency.

The contribution of the thyroarytenoid muscle is potentially more complex and may act to raise or lower fundamental frequency depending upon the degree of cricothyroid co-activation and the frequency range being produced (such as high or low pitch).

Visual Representation of the Classifications of Vocal Fold Layers

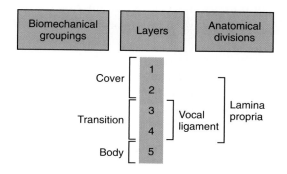

Blood Supply

The superior laryngeal branch (superior laryngeal artery) of the superior thyroid artery supplies the superior part of the larynx. The cricothyroid branch of the superior laryngeal artery supplies the cricothyroid cartilage. The inferior laryngeal branch of the inferior thyroid artery supplies the inferior part of the larynx.

Innervation

The laryngeal muscles and their associated structures are innervated by the following two branches of the vagus nerve* (cranial nerve X):
1. The internal branch of the superior laryngeal nerve is sensory for the mucous membrane of the larynx above the vocal folds. The external branch is motor for the cricothyroid muscle.
2. The recurrent laryngeal nerve provides motor innervation of all intrinsic laryngeal muscles, except for the cricothyroid muscle. It is sensory for the mucous membranes below the vocal folds.

The third branch, the pharyngeal nerve, innervates the muscles and mucous membranes of the pharynx and soft palate.

The term *recurrent* means "returns, goes back to its origin." The recurrent laryngeal nerves distribute widely (particularly on the left side) before returning back to provide motor innervation to laryngeal muscles. In their trajectory, the recurrent laryngeal nerves pass near many structures that make them vulnerable to disease and damage during surgical intervention.

---

*The name of the vagus nerve comes from the word vagabond, which is related to its large distribution.

■ MUSCLES OF THE LARYNX

The following two types of muscles affect laryngeal function:
1. The intrinsic muscles, which have their points of attachments within the skeletal framework of the larynx.
2. The extrinsic muscles, which have one point of attachment on the laryngeal structures and another attachment outside of the larynx.
These muscles are discussed primarily in terms of their impact on the vibratory characteristics of the vocal folds for phonation.

Intrinsic Muscles of the Larynx (Figure 2-6)

The intrinsic muscles of the larynx have their origin and insertion within the laryngeal structure. Five intrinsic muscles control the following:
- Adduction-abduction.
- Tension-relaxation of the vocal folds.
- With adduction, the vocal processes (and the attached vocal folds) are rotated medially and inferiorly; with abduction, the vocal processes are rotated superiorly and laterally.
   During phonation, the following two types of adjustment are made:
1. Variation of the medial compression or the degree of force by which the vocal folds are joined at the median line.
2. Variation of the longitudinal tension or degree of stretching of the vocal folds.

Thyroarytenoid Muscle

The thyroarytenoid, or vocalis, muscle forms the major mass of the vocal folds and, consequently, the major portion of the laryngeal "valve" that protects the airway and serves other primary biological functions as previously mentioned. Its anterior origin is the inner surface of the thyroid, below the notch and near the thyroid angle. The muscle courses posteriorly to insert on the arytenoid cartilage, from the vocal to the muscular processes. Medially, it extends to the vocal ligament. The thyroarytenoid muscle is sometimes divided into the following two functional parts:
1. Thyrovocalis: medial portion (sometimes named the vocal portion or vocalis muscle)
2. Thyromuscularis: lateral portion
Isolated, unopposed contraction of the thyroarytenoid shortens and thickens the body of the vocal folds but loosens the cover. The impact on fundamental frequency of vibration of the vocal folds depends upon the degree of co-contraction with the cricothyroid and the frequency range being produced, as discussed previously. Muscle shortening and increased mass may contribute to vocal fold adduction.

The thyroarytenoid muscle is innervated by the anterior division (also known as the *inferior laryngeal nerve*) of the recurrent laryngeal nerve.

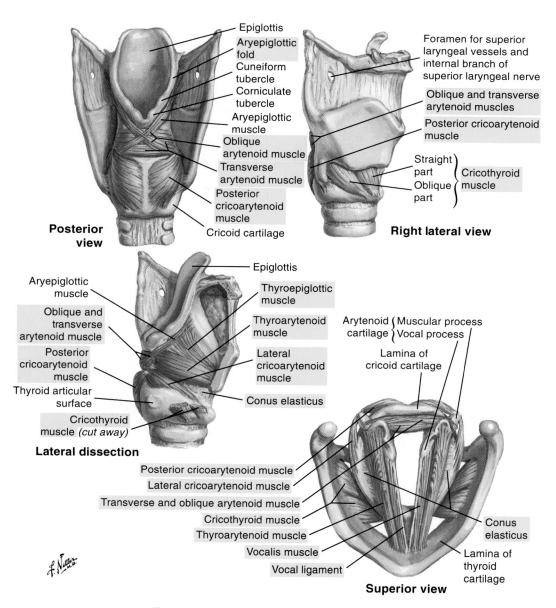

Posterior view

- Epiglottis
- Aryepiglottic fold
- Cuneiform tubercle
- Corniculate tubercle
- Aryepiglottic muscle
- Oblique arytenoid muscle
- Transverse arytenoid muscle
- Posterior cricoarytenoid muscle
- Cricoid cartilage

Right lateral view

- Foramen for superior laryngeal vessels and internal branch of superior laryngeal nerve
- Oblique and transverse arytenoid muscles
- Posterior cricoarytenoid muscle
- Straight part ⎱ Cricothyroid
- Oblique part ⎰ muscle

Lateral dissection

- Aryepiglottic muscle
- Oblique and transverse arytenoid muscle
- Posterior cricoarytenoid muscle
- Thyroid articular surface
- Cricothyroid muscle *(cut away)*
- Epiglottis
- Thyroepiglottic muscle
- Thyroarytenoid muscle
- Lateral cricoarytenoid muscle
- Conus elasticus

Superior view

- Arytenoid cartilage ⎱ Muscular process ⎰ Vocal process
- Lamina of cricoid cartilage
- Posterior cricoarytenoid muscle
- Lateral cricoarytenoid muscle
- Transverse and oblique arytenoid muscle
- Cricothyroid muscle
- Thyroarytenoid muscle
- Vocalis muscle
- Vocal ligament
- Conus elasticus
- Lamina of thyroid cartilage

Figure 2-6. The intrinsic muscles of the larynx.

Cricothyroid Muscle

The cricothyroid muscle is a major contributor to increasing vocal fold length and tension (vocal fold tensor) and may also assist in vocal fold abduction.

This muscle has the following two divisions:

1. The upper, more vertically directed portion (pars recta) courses from the anterior portion of the cricoid arch just lateral to the median line to the inferior surface of the thyroid cartilage.
2. The lower oblique portion (pars oblique) arises from the anterior portion of the cricoid arch (laterally to the median line) posteriorly and superiorly to insert on the inferior border of the inferior horn of the thyroid cartilage.

The exact actions of the two portions of the cricothyroid are controversial. The pars recta is thought to rotate the thyroid cartilage inferiorly, and the pars oblique is thought to pull the thyroid anteriorly. This increases the distance between the thyroid and arytenoid cartilages, and because of the attachment of the vocal folds between these two cartilages, increases the length and tension of the vocal folds.

The cricothyroid muscle is innervated by the external branch of the superior laryngeal nerve.

Posterior Cricoarytenoid Muscle

The posterior cricoarytenoid muscle is a fan-shaped muscle that is the only abductor muscle of the vocal folds. It arises from the posterior quadrate lamina of the cricoid, and fibers course superiorly and laterally to insert onto the posterior surface of the muscular process of the arytenoid. This muscle is often divided into medial and lateral bellies. Its action is to rotate the muscular processes downward and toward the midline, which moves the vocal processes laterally and superiorly, lengthening, elevating, and abducting the vocal folds.

The posterior cricoarytenoid muscle is innervated by the posterior branch of the recurrent laryngeal nerve.

Lateral Cricoarytenoid Muscle

The lateral cricoarytenoid muscle acts as a vocal fold adductor. It arises from the superior surface of the lateral border of the cricoid arch to head superiorly and posteriorly and to insert on the anterior portion of the muscular process of the arytenoids. Some fibers are continuous with those of the thyroarytenoid muscle. The contraction of the lateral cricoarytenoid muscle pulls on the muscular process and rotates the vocal processes toward the median line, which adducts the vocal folds.

The lateral cricoarytenoid muscle is innervated by the anterior division of the recurrent laryngeal nerve.

Interarytenoid (Arytenoid) Muscle

The interarytenoid (arytenoid) muscle is also an adductor muscle, with the following two parts:

1. The transverse portion is the deeper portion, with horizontally directed fibers from the lateral margin of one arytenoid to the lateral margin of the other.
2. The oblique portion is more superficial, with obliquely directed fibers from the apex of one arytenoid to the lateral portion of the base of the other. Some fibers continue superiorly as the aryepiglottic muscle.

The action of the interarytenoid muscle is to pull the two arytenoids together to the midline and thus adduct the vocal folds. The muscle is also involved in the regulation of medial compression between the vocal folds.

The interarytenoid is innervated by the anterior division of the recurrent laryngeal nerve.

Extrinsic Muscles of the Larynx (Figure 2-7)

All of the extrinsic muscles have one point of attachment on laryngeal structures or structures that influence laryngeal position and movement (e.g., the hyoid bone). They contribute to the suspension, support, and mobility of the larynx. Extrinsic laryngeal muscles are further classified by whether they are located above or below the hyoid bone.

Actions of the extrinsic muscles are classified in the following two basic groups:

1. Four infrahyoid muscles are sometimes classified as laryngeal "depressors."
2. Five suprahyoid muscles are sometimes classified as laryngeal "elevators."

Four Infrahyoid Muscles or Laryngeal Depressors

The function of the four infrahyoid muscles is to move the larynx downward, forward, or backward.

Thyrohyoid Muscle

The thyrohyoid muscle is located superficial to the superior portion of the sternohyoid muscle. It courses from the oblique line of the thyroid cartilage to the greater horn of the hyoid bone. Contraction of the thyrohyoid muscle approximates the thyroid cartilage and hyoid bone. Depending on which point of attachment is most mobile and the simultaneous activation of other muscles, the thyrohyoid muscle can pull down on the hyoid bone or lift the thyroid cartilage. Thus this muscle can be classified as either a laryngeal elevator or depressor. The thyrohyoid muscle is also important for laryngeal elevation for swallowing.

Sternohyoid Muscle

The sternohyoid muscle courses from the sternum to the hyoid bone. It can pull down on the hyoid bone and, with it, the larynx.

Omohyoid Muscle

The omohyoid muscle is a two-bellied muscle (inferior and superior) that extends from the scapula through an intermediate tendon to the hyoid bone. Contraction can pull down on the hyoid bone.

Sternothyroid Muscle

The sternothyroid muscle is located superficial to the sternohyoid muscle and courses from the sternum and first costal cartilage to the oblique line of the thyroid. Contraction of this muscle results in downward movement of the thyroid. It also may shorten the vocal folds, decreasing tension and frequency of vibration.

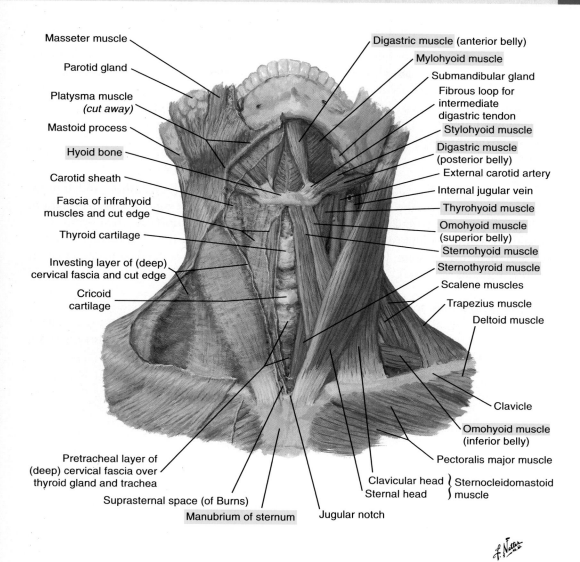

Masseter muscle

Parotid gland

Platysma muscle
(cut away)

Mastoid process

Hyoid bone

Carotid sheath

Fascia of infrahyoid
muscles and cut edge

Thyroid cartilage

Investing layer of (deep)
cervical fascia and cut edge

Cricoid
cartilage

Pretracheal layer of
(deep) cervical fascia over
thyroid gland and trachea

Suprasternal space (of Burns)

Manubrium of sternum

Digastric muscle (anterior belly)

Mylohyoid muscle

Submandibular gland

Fibrous loop for
intermediate
digastric tendon

Stylohyoid muscle

Digastric muscle
(posterior belly)

External carotid artery

Internal jugular vein

Thyrohyoid muscle

Omohyoid muscle
(superior belly)

Sternohyoid muscle

Sternothyroid muscle

Scalene muscles

Trapezius muscle

Deltoid muscle

Clavicle

Omohyoid muscle
(inferior belly)

Pectoralis major muscle

Clavicular head ⎱ Sternocleidomastoid
Sternal head ⎰ muscle

Jugular notch

Figure 2-7. An anterior view of the muscles of the neck. Note the four infrahyoid muscles:
(1) thyrohyoid, (2) sternohyoid, (3) omohyoid, and (4) sternothyroid.

Five Suprahyoid Muscles or Laryngeal Elevators (Figure 2-8)

The function of the five suprahyoid muscles is to open the mouth by pulling down on the mandible, elevating the hyoid bone, and moving the larynx upward, forward, or backward.

The five muscles are as follows:

1. Digastric muscle
2. Mylohyoid muscle
3. Geniohyoid muscle
4. Stylohyoid muscle
5. Hyoglossus muscle

These muscles all have a point of attachment on the skull or the mandible and another point of attachment on the hyoid bone. Because they play important roles in mastication, swallowing, and the articulatory movements of speech production, the mylohyoid, geniohyoid, digastric, genioglossus, and hyoglossus muscles are examined in further detail in Part 3: Articulatory System, p. 105–167. The stylohyoid muscle is detailed in the table on extrinsic muscles on p. 100.

Cricopharyngeal Muscle

The cricopharyngeal is part of the inferior constrictor muscle forming a portion of the pharynx. It plays an important role in swallowing (see Part 3: Articulatory System, p. 105–167). Contraction of this muscle may also influence vocal fold length.

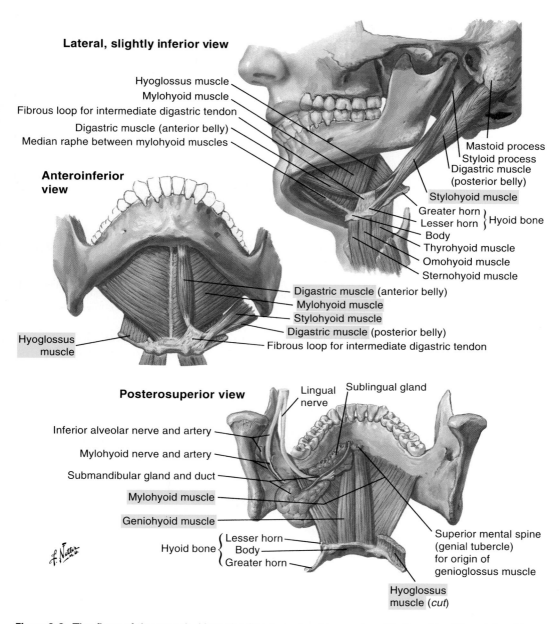

Lateral, slightly inferior view

Hyoglossus muscle
Mylohyoid muscle
Fibrous loop for intermediate digastric tendon
Digastric muscle (anterior belly)
Median raphe between mylohyoid muscles

Mastoid process
Styloid process
Digastric muscle (posterior belly)
Stylohyoid muscle
Greater horn }
Lesser horn } Hyoid bone
Body
Thyrohyoid muscle
Omohyoid muscle
Sternohyoid muscle

Anteroinferior view

Digastric muscle (anterior belly)
Mylohyoid muscle
Stylohyoid muscle
Digastric muscle (posterior belly)
Fibrous loop for intermediate digastric tendon

Hyoglossus muscle

Posterosuperior view

Lingual nerve   Sublingual gland

Inferior alveolar nerve and artery
Mylohyoid nerve and artery
Submandibular gland and duct
Mylohyoid muscle
Geniohyoid muscle

Hyoid bone { Lesser horn
Body
Greater horn

Superior mental spine (genial tubercle) for origin of genioglossus muscle

Hyoglossus muscle (cut)

Figure 2-8. The floor of the mouth. Note the five suprahyoid muscles: (1) digastric, (2) mylohyoid, (3) geniohyoid, (4) stylohyoid, and (5) hyoglossus.

Intrinsic Muscles of the Larynx (see Figures 2-3 and 2-6, pp. 85 and 91)		
Muscle(s)	**Description**	**Origin**
Thyroarytenoid, or vocalis, muscle	Muscle fibers contributing to the vocal folds	Anteriorly from the inner surface of the thyroid
Cricothyroid	Fan-shaped muscle located between the cricoid and the thyroid cartilages, with two divisions: (1) pars oblique and (2) pars recta	Cricoid arch
Posterior cricoarytenoid	Fan-shaped muscle on the posterior surface of cricoid	Quadrate lamina of the cricoid
Lateral cricoarytenoid	Located deep to the thyroid cartilage	Superior surface of the anterolateral border of the cricoid arch
Interarytenoid	Nonpaired muscle composed of fibers oriented in oblique and transverse direction. Oblique fibers cross between the arytenoids to form an X and are located superficial to the transverse fibers.	**Oblique fibers** Base of one arytenoid Continuous with aryepiglottic muscle fibers **Transverse fibers** On the lateral border of each arytenoid between the muscular processes and the apex

Intrinsic Muscles of the Larynx, cont'd

Insertion	Action	Motor Innervation
Vocal and muscular processes of the vocal folds	May function to increase *or* decrease fundamental frequency depending upon the co-activation of other intrinsic muscles such as the cricothyroid	Recurrent laryngeal nerve of the vagus (cranial nerve X)
Inferior border of the lamina and inferior cornu of the thyroid	Decreases the distance between the thyroid and the cricoid Pulls thyroid anteriorly, lengthening and thinning the vocal folds and increasing longitudinal tension and pitch (tensor)	External branch of the superior laryngeal nerve of the vagus (cranial nerve X)
Posterior surface of the muscular process of the arytenoid	Abducts the arytenoids and opens the glottis (abductor)	Recurrent laryngeal nerve of the vagus (cranial nerve X)
Anterior surface of the muscular process of the arytenoid	Approximates the vocal processes, closing the glottis (adductor)	Recurrent laryngeal nerve of the vagus (cranial nerve X).
Oblique fibers Apex of the opposite arytenoid **Transverse fibers** Lateral border of the opposite arytenoid	Approximates the arytenoids and closes the glottis (adductor)	Recurrent laryngeal nerve of the vagus (cranial nerve X)

Extrinsic Muscles of the Larynx (Suprahyoid Muscles)

Muscle(s)	Description	Origin	Insertion	Action	Innervation
Digastric (Figure 2-9, p. 102 ; see also Figure 2-8, p. 97)	Anterior and posterior bellies linked by a tendon attached to the body and greater horn of the hyoid bone	**Posterior belly** Mastoid process **Anterior belly** Internal surface of mandible, near midline	**Posterior belly** Intermediate tendon **Anterior belly** Intermediate tendon	**Posterior belly** With the mandible stabilized, the posterior belly elevates and retracts the hyoid. **Anterior belly** With the hyoid fixed by the infrahyoid and suprahyoid muscles, the digastric opens the jaw.	**Posterior belly** Digastric branch of the facial nerve (cranial nerve VII) **Anterior belly** Mylohyoid branch of the inferior alveolar nerve of the mandibular branch of the trigeminal (cranial nerve V)
Mylohyoid (Figure 2-10, p. 103; see also Figure 2-8, p. 97)	Thin muscle forming the muscular "floor" of the oral cavity Deep to the digastric	Mylohyoid line on the internal surface of the mandible	**Posterior fibers** Body of the hyoid bone **Anterior fibers** Linked with fibers of the opposite side through the median raphe	Pulls hyoid superiorly and anteriorly	Mylohyoid branch of the inferior alveolar nerve of the mandibular branch of the trigeminal (cranial nerve V)
Geniohyoid (see Figures 2-8 and 2-10, pp. 97 and 103)	Narrow, cylindrically shaped muscle deep to the mylohyoid	Inferior mental spine (genial tubercle) on the internal surface of the mandible	Anterior surface of the body of the hyoid	Pulls hyoid anteriorly	First cervical spinal nerve (C1) traveling with fibers of the hypoglossal nerve (cranial nerve XII)
Stylohyoid (see Figures 2-8 and 2-10, pp. 97 and 103)	Long, thin muscle roughly parallel to the posterior belly of the digastric	Styloid process of the temporal bone	Body of the hyoid bone near the greater horn	Elevates and retracts the hyoid bone	Stylohyoid branch of the facial nerve (cranial nerve VII)
Hyoglossus (see Figure 2-10, p. 103)	Thin muscle from the hyoid to the tongue	Body and greater horn of the hyoid	Side of the tongue medial to styloglossus	Pulls the hyoid superiorly and depresses the back of the tongue	Hyoglossal branch of the hypoglossal nerve (cranial nerve XII)

Extrinsic Muscles of the Larynx (Infrahyoid Muscles) (see Figure 2-9, p. 104)

Muscle(s)	Description	Origin	Insertion	Action	Innervation
Thyrohyoid	Thin muscle that appears as a continuation of sternohyoid muscle	Oblique line of the thyroid cartilage	On the inferior side of the body and the greater horn of hyoid bone	Lowers the hyoid or elevates the thyroid	First cervical spinal nerve (C1) traveling with fibers of the hypoglossal nerve (cranial nerve XII)
Sternohyoid	Thin muscle on the anterior surface of the neck	Posterior surface of the manubrium and medial border of the clavicle	Inferior border of the body of the hyoid bone	Lowers the hyoid and the larynx	Cervical spinal nerves C1–C3 via ansa cervicalis
Omohyoid	Thin, narrow muscle, with superior and inferior portions joined by a central tendon connected by fascia to the clavicle	**Inferior belly** Superior border of the scapula **Superior belly** Intermediate tendon	**Inferior belly** Intermediate tendon **Superior belly** Inferior border of the body of the hyoid	Depresses the hyoid	**Inferior belly** Cervical spinal nerves C1–C3 via ansa cervicalis **Posterior belly** First cervical spinal nerve (C1) via the superior ramus of the ansa cervicalis
Sternothyroid	Long, thin muscle on the anterior surface of the neck	Posterior surface of the manubrium of the sternum and the first costal cartilage	Oblique line of the thyroid cartilage	Lowers the thyroid cartilage and the larynx	Cervical spinal nerves C1–C3 via ansa cervicalis

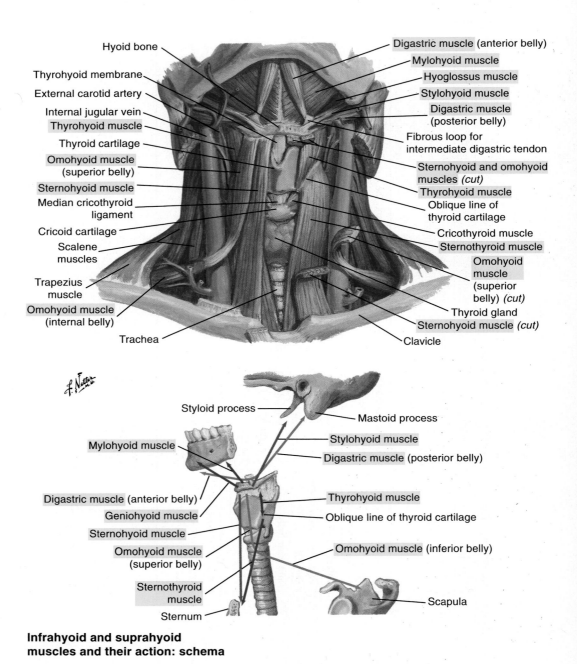

Hyoid bone

Thyrohyoid membrane

External carotid artery

Internal jugular vein

Thyrohyoid muscle

Thyroid cartilage

Omohyoid muscle (superior belly)

Sternohyoid muscle

Median cricothyroid ligament

Cricoid cartilage

Scalene muscles

Trapezius muscle

Omohyoid muscle (internal belly)

Trachea

Digastric muscle (anterior belly)

Mylohyoid muscle

Hyoglossus muscle

Stylohyoid muscle

Digastric muscle (posterior belly)

Fibrous loop for intermediate digastric tendon

Sternohyoid and omohyoid muscles (cut)

Thyrohyoid muscle

Oblique line of thyroid cartilage

Cricothyroid muscle

Sternothyroid muscle

Omohyoid muscle (superior belly) (cut)

Thyroid gland

Sternohyoid muscle (cut)

Clavicle

Styloid process

Mastoid process

Mylohyoid muscle

Stylohyoid muscle

Digastric muscle (posterior belly)

Digastric muscle (anterior belly)

Geniohyoid muscle

Sternohyoid muscle

Omohyoid muscle (superior belly)

Sternothyroid muscle

Sternum

Thyrohyoid muscle

Oblique line of thyroid cartilage

Omohyoid muscle (inferior belly)

Scapula

Infrahyoid and suprahyoid muscles and their action: schema

Figure 2-9. The infrahyoid and suprahyoid muscles and their actions.

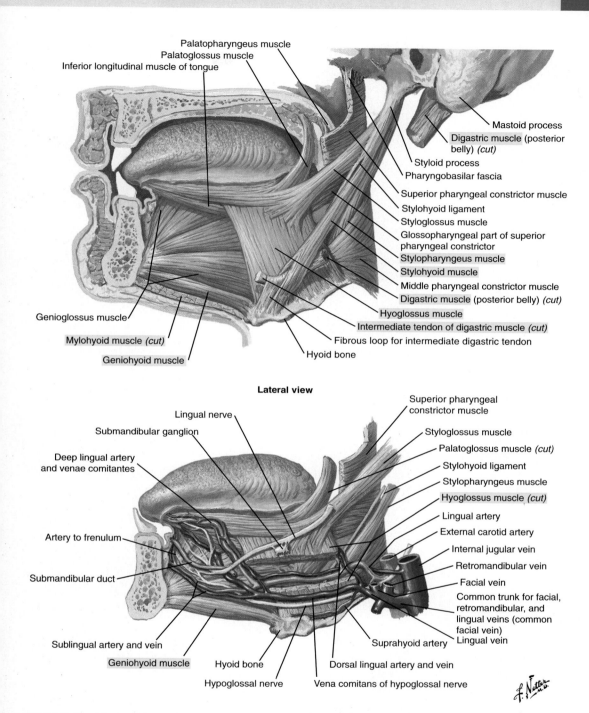

Palatopharyngeus muscle
Palatoglossus muscle
Inferior longitudinal muscle of tongue

Mastoid process
Digastric muscle (posterior belly) *(cut)*
Styloid process
Pharyngobasilar fascia
Superior pharyngeal constrictor muscle
Stylohyoid ligament
Styloglossus muscle
Glossopharyngeal part of superior pharyngeal constrictor
Stylopharyngeus muscle
Stylohyoid muscle
Middle pharyngeal constrictor muscle
Digastric muscle (posterior belly) *(cut)*
Hyoglossus muscle
Intermediate tendon of digastric muscle *(cut)*
Fibrous loop for intermediate digastric tendon
Hyoid bone

Genioglossus muscle
Mylohyoid muscle *(cut)*
Geniohyoid muscle

Lateral view

Lingual nerve
Submandibular ganglion
Deep lingual artery and venae comitantes

Superior pharyngeal constrictor muscle
Styloglossus muscle
Palatoglossus muscle *(cut)*
Stylohyoid ligament
Stylopharyngeus muscle
Hyoglossus muscle *(cut)*
Lingual artery
External carotid artery
Internal jugular vein
Retromandibular vein
Facial vein
Common trunk for facial, retromandibular, and lingual veins (common facial vein)
Lingual vein

Artery to frenulum
Submandibular duct

Sublingual artery and vein
Geniohyoid muscle
Hyoid bone
Hypoglossal nerve
Dorsal lingual artery and vein
Vena comitans of hypoglossal nerve
Suprahyoid artery

f. Netter. m.d.

Figure 2-10. A lateral view of the tongue and surrounding muscles. Note the extrinsic muscles of the larynx.

ARTICULATORY SYSTEM

3

■ OVERVIEW

The supralaryngeal vocal tract is crucial for speech sound generation. Its function is to modify the laryngeal sound source to produce the sounds of speech. Vowels are created by changing the configuration of the vocal tract, which acts as a filter with modifiable resonant modes. Frequencies at or near these resonant modes (called *formant frequencies*) pass most effectively, whereas others are attenuated. Consequently, the frequency spectrum of the sound generated by the vibrating vocal folds is modified as it passes through the filter. The filter characteristics of the upper vocal tract depend on its shape, which is modified by movements of the articulators (e.g., tongue, jaw, and lips) through muscular action.

Consonants are more complex and require rapid movements of one or more of the speech articulators to create transient or turbulent sound sources and may include an additional sound source from the vibrating vocal folds for voiced consonants. The same oral-articulatory structures that participate in speech production are also vital for the manipulation and movement of food and liquids during mastication and swallowing.

This section focuses on a study of the articulatory system. First, cranial anatomy relative to the articulators and other associated structures of the vocal tract is discussed, followed by an examination of the various muscles of articulation and their respective functions.

■ CRANIAL ANATOMY

The skull is an extremely complex osseous structure that provides protection for the brain (and middle and inner ears) and is the point of attachment of many muscles important for speech, mastication, and swallowing. The skull is composed of 22 bones (excluding the 6 middle ear ossicles), 8 paired and 6 unpaired. They are joined together by sutures, which provide for growth in the developing skull, except for the mandible or lower jaw, which is the only movable cranial bone. In fact, the skull is sometimes divided into the cranium (which includes the facial skeleton) and the mandible. The cranium can be further divided into the *cranial vault,* the upper bowl-like portion that includes the skullcap or calvaria, and the *cranial base.* We will use the following main divisions of the skull:

1. The cranium (cranial skeleton), which is located in the superoposterior quadrant of the skull
2. The facial skeleton (including the mandible), which is located in the anteroinferior quadrant of the skull

Cranium (Figures 3-1, 3-2 [p. 110], and 3-3 [p. 111])

The cranium contains eight bones, four of which are unpaired.

Unpaired Bones

- The frontal bone contributes to the forehead, the anterior internal surface of the skull, the anterior cranial fossa, the orbits, and the nasal cavity.
- The occipital bone forms the posteroinferior margin of the cranial cavity and contributes to the posterior cranial fossa. It encloses the foramen magnum, which is the point of communication between the brain and spinal cord.
- The sphenoid bone forms the pterygoid fossa located between the medial and lateral pterygoid plates. It contributes to the anterior and middle cranial fossae, the orbit, the temporal fossa, the infratemporal fossa, the pterygoid palatine fossa, the scaphoid fossa, the nasal cavity, and the lateral wall of the cranial vault.
- The ethmoid bone contributes to the anterior cranial fossa, the lateral and superior walls of the nasal cavity, the nasal septum, and the medial wall of the orbital cavity.

Paired Bones

- Temporal bones contribute to the inferolateral margins of the cranial vault. They form the posterolateral part of the middle cranial fossa and the anterolateral part of the posterior cranial fossa and contain the middle and inner ear.
- Parietal bones contribute to the superior, lateral, and posterior portions of the cranial vault.

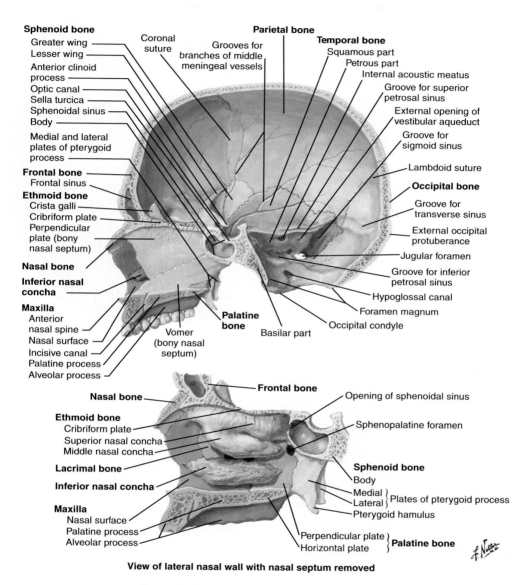

Sphenoid bone
- Greater wing
- Lesser wing
- Anterior clinoid process
- Optic canal
- Sella turcica
- Sphenoidal sinus
- Body
- Medial and lateral plates of pterygoid process

Frontal bone
- Frontal sinus

Ethmoid bone
- Crista galli
- Cribriform plate
- Perpendicular plate (bony nasal septum)

Nasal bone

Inferior nasal concha

Maxilla
- Anterior nasal spine
- Nasal surface
- Incisive canal
- Palatine process
- Alveolar process

Coronal suture

Grooves for branches of middle meningeal vessels

Vomer (bony nasal septum)

Palatine bone

Basilar part

Parietal bone

Temporal bone
- Squamous part
- Petrous part
- Internal acoustic meatus
- Groove for superior petrosal sinus
- External opening of vestibular aqueduct
- Groove for sigmoid sinus

Lambdoid suture

Occipital bone
- Groove for transverse sinus
- External occipital protuberance

Jugular foramen

Groove for inferior petrosal sinus

Hypoglossal canal

Foramen magnum

Occipital condyle

Frontal bone

Nasal bone

Ethmoid bone
- Cribriform plate
- Superior nasal concha
- Middle nasal concha

Lacrimal bone

Inferior nasal concha

Maxilla
- Nasal surface
- Palatine process
- Alveolar process

Opening of sphenoidal sinus

Sphenopalatine foramen

Sphenoid bone
- Body
- Medial ⎫
- Lateral ⎭ Plates of pterygoid process
- Pterygoid hamulus

Perpendicular plate ⎫
Horizontal plate ⎭ **Palatine bone**

View of lateral nasal wall with nasal septum removed

Figure 3-1. A midsagittal section of the cranium.

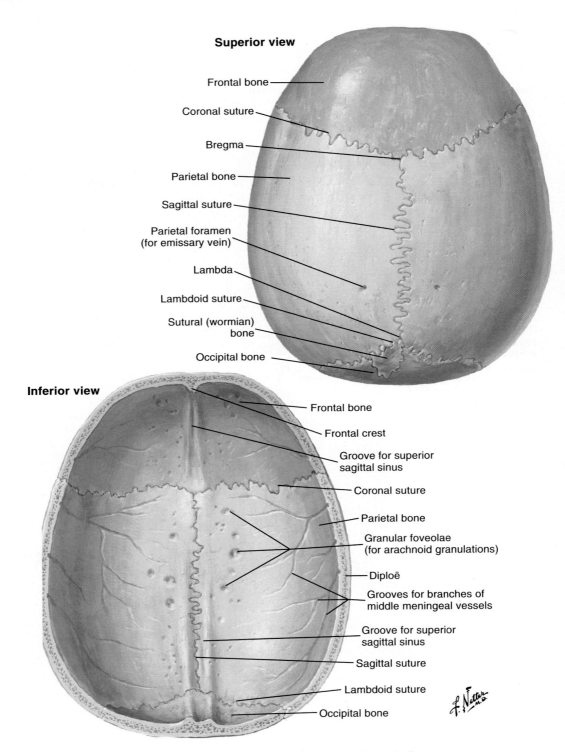

Superior view

Frontal bone

Coronal suture

Bregma

Parietal bone

Sagittal suture

Parietal foramen
(for emissary vein)

Lambda

Lambdoid suture

Sutural (wormian)
bone

Occipital bone

Inferior view

Frontal bone

Frontal crest

Groove for superior
sagittal sinus

Coronal suture

Parietal bone

Granular foveolae
(for arachnoid granulations)

Diploë

Grooves for branches of
middle meningeal vessels

Groove for superior
sagittal sinus

Sagittal suture

Lambdoid suture

Occipital bone

Figure 3-2. Superior and inferior views of the skullcap.

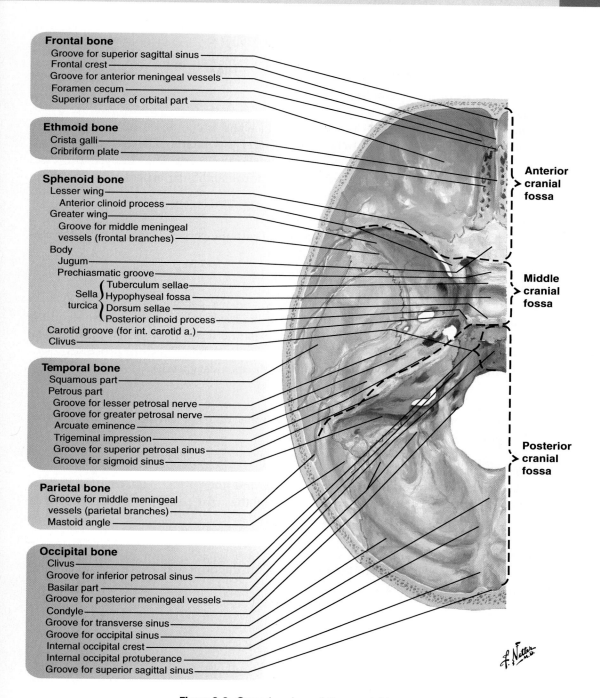

Frontal bone
- Groove for superior sagittal sinus
- Frontal crest
- Groove for anterior meningeal vessels
- Foramen cecum
- Superior surface of orbital part

Ethmoid bone
- Crista galli
- Cribriform plate

Sphenoid bone
- Lesser wing
- Anterior clinoid process
- Greater wing
- Groove for middle meningeal vessels (frontal branches)
- Body
- Jugum
- Prechiasmatic groove
- Sella turcica
  - Tuberculum sellae
  - Hypophyseal fossa
  - Dorsum sellae
  - Posterior clinoid process
- Carotid groove (for int. carotid a.)
- Clivus

Temporal bone
- Squamous part
- Petrous part
- Groove for lesser petrosal nerve
- Groove for greater petrosal nerve
- Arcuate eminence
- Trigeminal impression
- Groove for superior petrosal sinus
- Groove for sigmoid sinus

Parietal bone
- Groove for middle meningeal vessels (parietal branches)
- Mastoid angle

Occipital bone
- Clivus
- Groove for inferior petrosal sinus
- Basilar part
- Groove for posterior meningeal vessels
- Condyle
- Groove for transverse sinus
- Groove for occipital sinus
- Internal occipital crest
- Internal occipital protuberance
- Groove for superior sagittal sinus

Anterior
cranial
fossa

Middle
cranial
fossa

Posterior
cranial
fossa

Figure 3-3. Superior view of the cranial base.

Facial Skeleton (Figures 3-4, 3-5 [p. 114], and 3-6 [p. 115])

The facial skeleton is constructed of 14 bones, two of which are unpaired.

Unpaired Bones of the Facial Skeleton
Mandible
The mandible forms the inferior border of the face and is composed of three parts: the horizontal body containing the alveolar process and the mandibular teeth and the two rami. On each ramus are the coronoid and condylar processes. The condylar processes articulate with the cranial temporal bones by temporomandibular articulations that form the temporomandibular joint.

Vomer
The vomer forms part of the boney nasal septum (with the perpendicular plate of the ethmoid) and the posterior wall of the nasal cavity.

Paired Bones of the Facial Skeleton
Maxilla
The maxilla is made up of two bones that join at the median line. They contribute to the upper jaw, cheek, infratemporal region, pterygopalatine fossa, floor of the orbit, palatal vault, and lateral walls and floor of the nasal cavities. Each bone has four processes: zygomatic, frontal, palatine, and alveolar (supporting the maxillary teeth).

Nasal Bones
Nasal bones contribute to the top and lateral walls of nasal cavities and the external "bridge" of the nose.

Palatine Bones
The palatine bones contribute to the lateral walls and floor of the nasal cavities, the oral cavity (more precisely the posterior one-third of the hard palate), the pterygopalatine fossa, and the posterior wall of the orbit.

Lacrimal Bones
The lacrimal bones contribute to the medial wall of the orbit and the lateral walls of the nasal cavities.

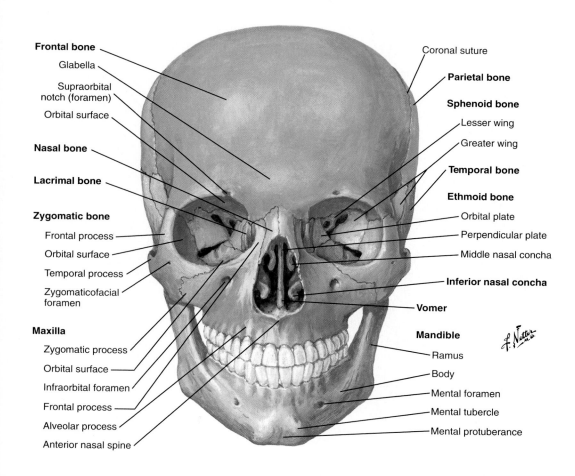

Frontal bone
Glabella
Supraorbital notch (foramen)
Orbital surface

Nasal bone

Lacrimal bone

Zygomatic bone
Frontal process
Orbital surface
Temporal process
Zygomaticofacial foramen

Maxilla
Zygomatic process
Orbital surface
Infraorbital foramen
Frontal process
Alveolar process
Anterior nasal spine

Coronal suture
Parietal bone
Sphenoid bone
Lesser wing
Greater wing
Temporal bone
Ethmoid bone
Orbital plate
Perpendicular plate
Middle nasal concha
Inferior nasal concha
Vomer
Mandible
Ramus
Body
Mental foramen
Mental tubercle
Mental protuberance

f. Netter

Right orbit: frontal and slightly lateral view

Orbital surface of frontal bone
Orbital surface of lesser wing of sphenoid bone
Superior orbital fissure
Optic canal (foramen)
Orbital surface of greater wing of sphenoid bone
Orbital surface of zygomatic bone
Inferior orbital fissure
Infraorbital groove

Posterior and Anterior ethmoidal foramina
Orbital plate of ethmoid bone
Lacrimal bone
Fossa for lacrimal sac
Orbital process of palatine bone
Orbital surface of maxilla

Figure 3-4. Anterior view of the skull and the facial skeleton.

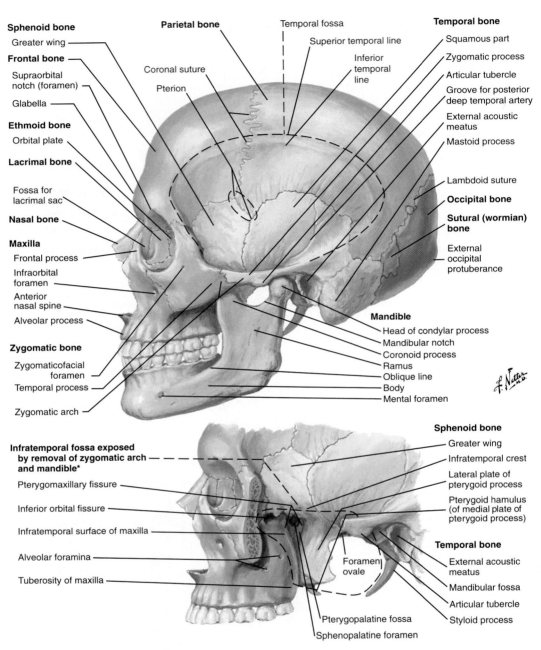

Sphenoid bone
Greater wing

Frontal bone
Supraorbital notch (foramen)
Glabella

Ethmoid bone
Orbital plate

Lacrimal bone

Fossa for lacrimal sac

Nasal bone

Maxilla
Frontal process
Infraorbital foramen
Anterior nasal spine
Alveolar process

Zygomatic bone

Zygomaticofacial foramen
Temporal process

Zygomatic arch

Parietal bone
Coronal suture
Pterion

Temporal fossa
Superior temporal line
Inferior temporal line

Temporal bone
Squamous part
Zygomatic process
Articular tubercle
Groove for posterior deep temporal artery
External acoustic meatus
Mastoid process

Lambdoid suture
Occipital bone
Sutural (wormian) bone
External occipital protuberance

Mandible
Head of condylar process
Mandibular notch
Coronoid process
Ramus
Oblique line
Body
Mental foramen

Infratemporal fossa exposed by removal of zygomatic arch and mandible*
Pterygomaxillary fissure
Inferior orbital fissure
Infratemporal surface of maxilla
Alveolar foramina
Tuberosity of maxilla

Sphenoid bone
Greater wing
Infratemporal crest
Lateral plate of pterygoid process
Pterygoid hamulus (of medial plate of pterygoid process)

Temporal bone
External acoustic meatus
Mandibular fossa
Articular tubercle
Styloid process

Foramen ovale
Pterygopalatine fossa
Sphenopalatine foramen

*Superficially, mastoid process forms posterior boundary.

Figure 3-5. Lateral view of the skull and the facial skeleton.

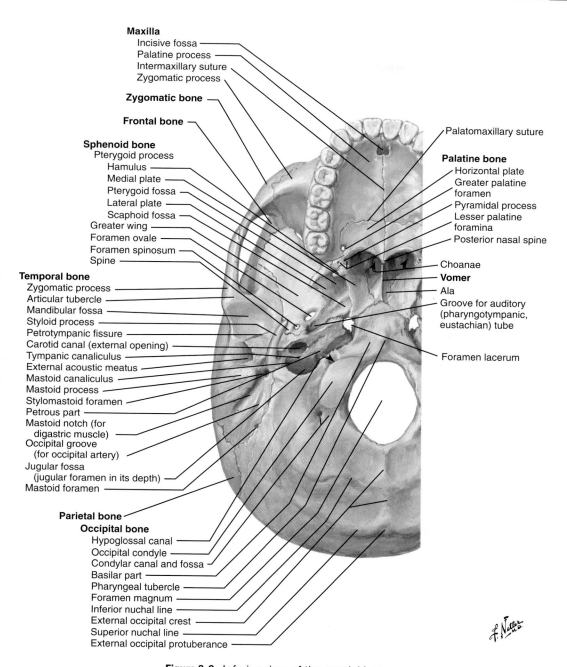

Maxilla
Incisive fossa
Palatine process
Intermaxillary suture
Zygomatic process

Zygomatic bone

Frontal bone

Sphenoid bone
Pterygoid process
Hamulus
Medial plate
Pterygoid fossa
Lateral plate
Scaphoid fossa
Greater wing
Foramen ovale
Foramen spinosum
Spine

Temporal bone
Zygomatic process
Articular tubercle
Mandibular fossa
Styloid process
Petrotympanic fissure
Carotid canal (external opening)
Tympanic canaliculus
External acoustic meatus
Mastoid canaliculus
Mastoid process
Stylomastoid foramen
Petrous part
Mastoid notch (for
digastric muscle)
Occipital groove
(for occipital artery)
Jugular fossa
(jugular foramen in its depth)
Mastoid foramen

Parietal bone
Occipital bone
Hypoglossal canal
Occipital condyle
Condylar canal and fossa
Basilar part
Pharyngeal tubercle
Foramen magnum
Inferior nuchal line
External occipital crest
Superior nuchal line
External occipital protuberance

Palatomaxillary suture

Palatine bone
Horizontal plate
Greater palatine
foramen
Pyramidal process
Lesser palatine
foramina
Posterior nasal spine

Choanae
Vomer
Ala
Groove for auditory
(pharyngotympanic,
eustachian) tube

Foramen lacerum

Figure 3-6. Inferior view of the cranial base.

Zygomatic Bones

The zygomatic bones form the skeletal support of the cheeks (thus the common name "cheekbone"). They contribute to the zygomatic arch, the lateral wall of the orbit, and the anterior wall of the infratemporal region.

Inferior Nasal Conchae

The inferior nasal conchae contribute to the formation of the lateral walls of the nasal cavities and the medial walls of the maxillary sinus.

Sinuses

Cranial and facial bones contain sinuses, which are air-filled cavities located near the nasal cavities, and are as follows:

- Maxillary sinus
- Frontal sinus
- Sphenoid sinus
- Ethmoid sinus

◼ VOCAL TRACT

The vocal tract is the portion of the upper airway above the vocal folds and is composed of the pharyngeal, nasal, and oral cavities.

Pharyngeal Cavity (Figures 3-7 and 3-8, pp. 118-119)

The pharyngeal cavity is made of the following three parts:
1. Nasopharynx
2. Oropharynx
3. Laryngopharynx

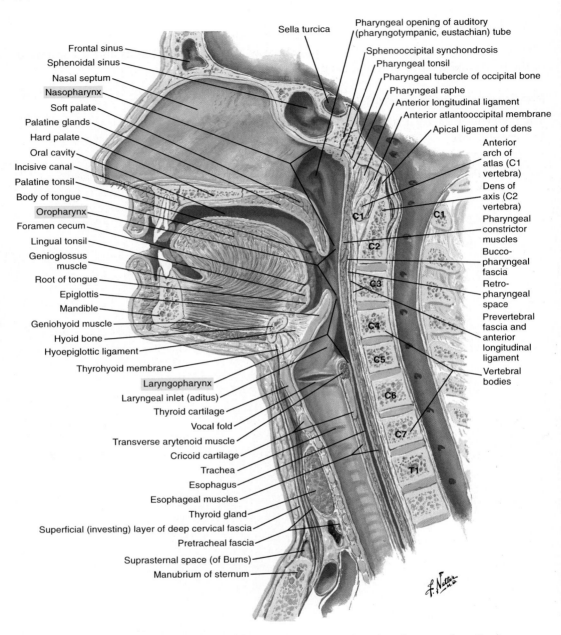

Figure 3-7. Median section of the head and neck. Note the pharyngeal cavity and associated structures.

Legends and labels of certain figures are highlighted in yellow to emphasize the related elements in the corresponding text.

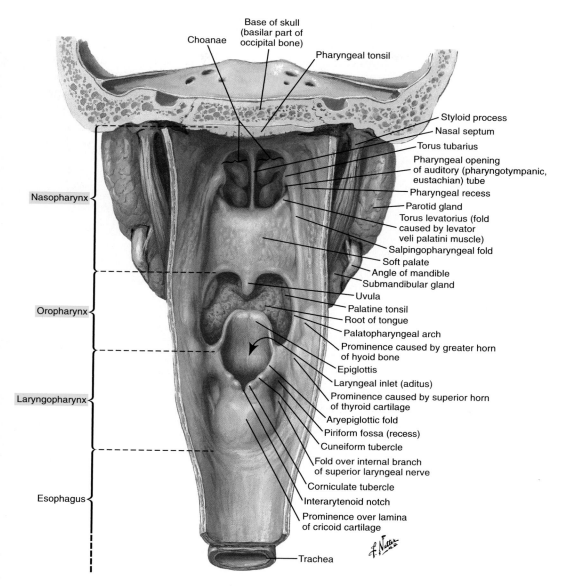

Choanae

Base of skull
(basilar part of
occipital bone)

Pharyngeal tonsil

Styloid process

Nasal septum

Torus tubarius

Pharyngeal opening
of auditory (pharyngotympanic,
eustachian) tube

Pharyngeal recess

Parotid gland

Torus levatorius (fold
caused by levator
veli palatini muscle)

Salpingopharyngeal fold

Soft palate

Angle of mandible

Submandibular gland

Uvula

Palatine tonsil

Root of tongue

Palatopharyngeal arch

Prominence caused by greater horn
of hyoid bone

Epiglottis

Laryngeal inlet (aditus)

Prominence caused by superior horn
of thyroid cartilage

Aryepiglottic fold

Piriform fossa (recess)

Cuneiform tubercle

Fold over internal branch
of superior laryngeal nerve

Corniculate tubercle

Interarytenoid notch

Prominence over lamina
of cricoid cartilage

Nasopharynx

Oropharynx

Laryngopharynx

Esophagus

Trachea

Figure 3-8. Opened posterior view of the pharynx.

Nasal Cavities (Figure 3-9)

The nasal cavities are divided medially by the nasal septum. The lateral walls are delineated by coiled, bony structures called *conchae* that are covered with mucous membranes. There are three conchae on each side: the superior, middle, and inferior nasal conchae. The conchae filter, moisten, and warm respired air. These convoluted structures increase surface area contact with the air.

During speech, except for the production of nasal sounds, the nasal cavities are isolated from the rest of the vocal tract by action of the velopharyngeal mechanism (see next section). The cartilages of the nasal cavities include the following:

- Septal cartilage
- Lateral cartilage
- Major alar cartilage
- Minor alar cartilage

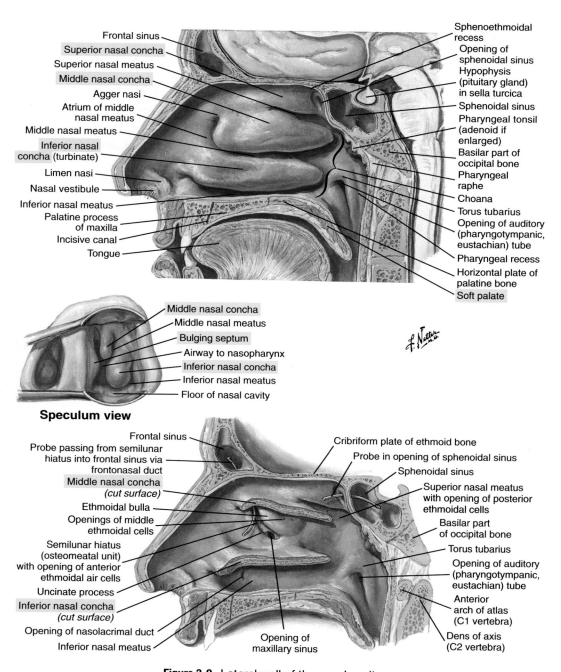

Speculum view

Figure 3-9. Lateral wall of the nasal cavity.

Oral Cavity (Figure 3-10)

Delineation of the oral cavity is as follows:
- Anterior limit is the lips and teeth.
- Lateral limit is the cheeks and teeth.
- Posterior limit is the palatoglossal arch.
- Superior limit is the palate.
- Inferior limit is the tongue and floor of the mouth.

Note that the delineation of the oral cavity varies considerably from one reference text to another.

The buccal space, or cavity, represents the space between the lips and the teeth and between the cheeks and the teeth. The articulators include the following (see Figure 3-10):
- Lips
- Cheeks
- Teeth
- Mandible
- Tongue
- Hard palate
- Soft palate
- Pharynx

During an examination of the oral cavity it is possible to see two pairs of folds located in the posterolateral part of the oral cavity, as follows:
1. The palatoglossal arch is formed by the palatoglossal muscle.
2. The palatopharyngeal arch is formed by the palatopharyngeus muscle.

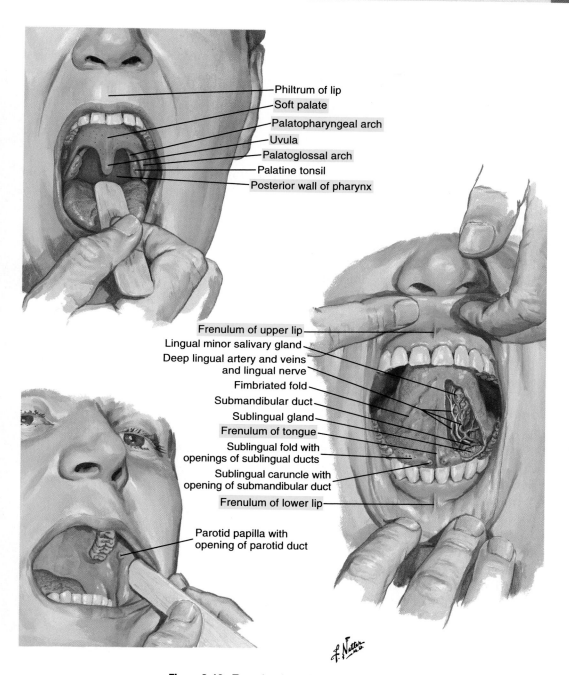

Philtrum of lip
Soft palate
Palatopharyngeal arch
Uvula
Palatoglossal arch
Palatine tonsil
Posterior wall of pharynx

Frenulum of upper lip
Lingual minor salivary gland
Deep lingual artery and veins
and lingual nerve
Fimbriated fold
Submandibular duct
Sublingual gland
Frenulum of tongue
Sublingual fold with
openings of sublingual ducts
Sublingual caruncle with
opening of submandibular duct
Frenulum of lower lip

Parotid papilla with
opening of parotid duct

Figure 3-10. Examination of the oral cavity.

Tonsils (see Figure 3-7, p. 118)

- Palatine tonsils, composed of lymphatic tissue, are located between the palatoglossal arch and the palatopharyngeal arch.
- Nasopharyngeal tonsils or pharyngeal tonsils (adenoids) are located on the posterior wall of the nasopharynx.
- Tubal tonsils are located near the opening of the auditory (pharyngotympanic, eustachian) tube.
- Lingual tonsils cover the base of the tongue.

Together, these tonsils form Waldeyer's tonsillar ring, which may protect the body from infections.

Palate (see Figure 3-7, p. 118)

The palate can be seen on the superior border of the oral cavity and is composed of the following:

- Hard palate is the osseous anterior two-thirds of the palate formed by the palatine processes of the maxilla (anteriorly) and the horizontal plates of the palatine bones (posteriorly).
- Soft palate or velum is a mobile structure forming the posterior one-third of the palate composed of connective tissue, muscular fibers, and mucosa.

At the posterior extremity of the palate, the uvula appears as an inferiorly directed projection of the posterior border of the soft palate.

Tongue (Figure 3-11)

The tongue is the primary articulator for speech sound production and is also crucial for the manipulation of food and liquid for mastication and swallowing. The following landmarks can be observed on the tongue surface:

- Foramen cecum
- Terminal sulcus
- Median sulcus
- Foliate, filiform, and fungiform papillae
- Lingual tonsils

When looking at the underside of the tongue, it is possible to see a bridge of tissue on the median line that links the tongue to the mouth floor. This fold is called the *lingual frenulum* (frenulum of the tongue) (see Figures 3-10 [p. 123] and 3-12 [p. 127]).

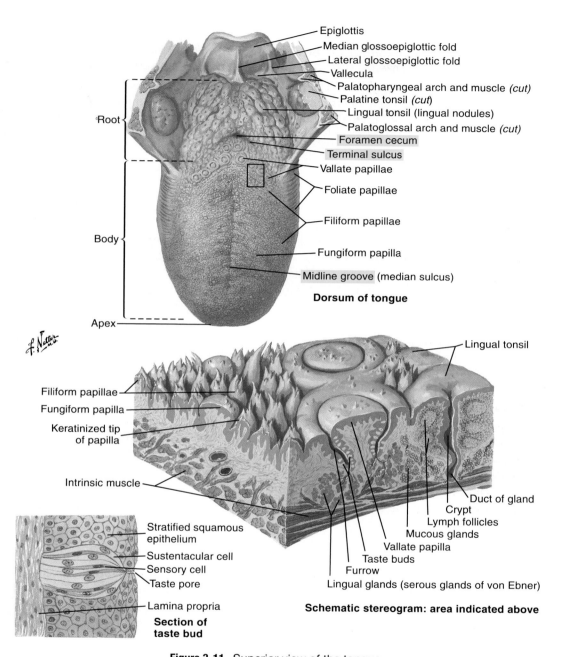

Epiglottis
Median glossoepiglottic fold
Lateral glossoepiglottic fold
Vallecula
Palatopharyngeal arch and muscle *(cut)*
Palatine tonsil *(cut)*
Lingual tonsil (lingual nodules)
Palatoglossal arch and muscle *(cut)*
Foramen cecum
Terminal sulcus
Vallate papillae
Foliate papillae
Filiform papillae
Fungiform papilla
Midline groove (median sulcus)

Root

Body

Apex

Dorsum of tongue

Lingual tonsil

Filiform papillae
Fungiform papilla
Keratinized tip
of papilla

Intrinsic muscle

Duct of gland
Crypt
Lymph follicles
Mucous glands
Vallate papilla
Taste buds
Furrow
Lingual glands (serous glands of von Ebner)

Stratified squamous
epithelium
Sustentacular cell
Sensory cell
Taste pore

Lamina propria
**Section of
taste bud**

Schematic stereogram: area indicated above

Figure 3-11. Superior view of the tongue.

Salivary Glands (Figure 3-12)

Saliva is extremely important for the breakdown and transport of food during mastication, taste, swallowing, and digestion. It is also crucial for oral health and as a lubricant for speech production and other oral motor activities. Saliva is produced by extrinsic and intrinsic salivary glands. There are three pairs of extrinsic salivary glands that produce the majority of the saliva. They are located outside but secrete into the oral cavity and are as follows:

1. Parotid glands
2. Submandibular glands
3. Sublingual glands

Lips (see Figure 3-10, p. 123)

The lips occupy the anterior extremity of the oral cavity and are important for speech sound production, mastication, and swallowing. The external surface of the lips is covered by skin and the internal surface by mucous membrane. The tissue between these two layers (external and internal) is muscular, adipose, and glandular.

Looking at the external surface of the lips, the following are visible (see Figure 3-10, p. 123):

- The nasolabial fold (and associated crease, furrow, or sulcus) is a prominent fold from the lateral margin of the nose to the angle of the mouth.
- The labiomandibular fold or "jowl" extends from the corner of the mouth to the mandible. It is often seen as a continuation of the more superior nasolabial fold. Facial muscle contraction and movements of the nasolabial and labiomandibular folds (and associated creases) signal important facial expressions such as smiling.
- Philtral ridges are the two vertical parallel crests above the superior lip.
- The philtrum is the space between the philtral ridges.
- The mentolabial sulcus is between the lower lip and the chin.
- Cupid's bow is the well-defined border of the upper lip.
- Vermilion zones are the transition zones between the skin of the face and the mucous membrane that covers the internal surface of the upper and lower lips.
- Labial commissure is the angle or corner of the mouth.
- The modiolus is not visible on surface inspection but is located lateral to the labial commissure. There is one on each side, and they are dense, mobile, roughly cone-shaped masses formed by the convergence of muscle fibers from several labial/facial muscles and other fibrous tissue. They are key anatomical structures for controlling movements of the lips for a variety of activities, including speech, mastication, swallowing, and facial expression.

The internal surface of the lips is covered by a mucous membrane with a thin and transparent epithelium. The pink color is due to underlying vascularity.

Pulling up on the upper lip exposes the frenulum of the upper lip, which is the median tissue that links the lip to the maxilla. Pulling down on the lower lip exposes the frenulum of the lower lip, which is a median fold of tissue that links the lower lip to the mandible.

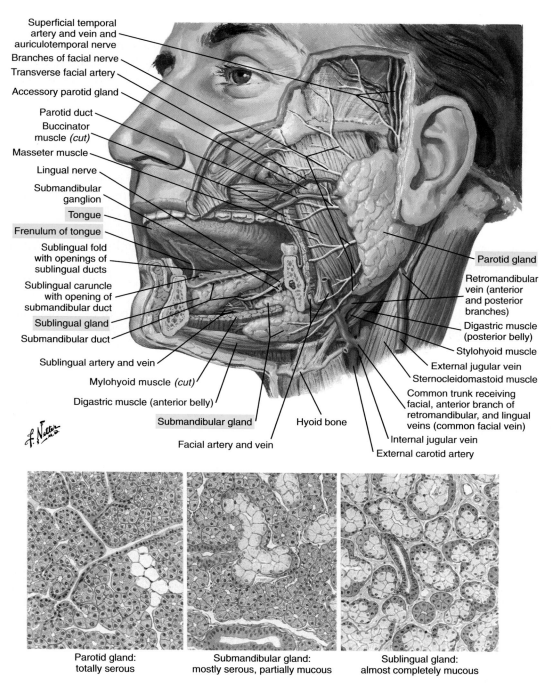

Superficial temporal artery and vein and auriculotemporal nerve
Branches of facial nerve
Transverse facial artery
Accessory parotid gland
Parotid duct
Buccinator muscle *(cut)*
Masseter muscle
Lingual nerve
Submandibular ganglion
Tongue
Frenulum of tongue
Sublingual fold with openings of sublingual ducts
Sublingual caruncle with opening of submandibular duct
Sublingual gland
Submandibular duct
Sublingual artery and vein
Mylohyoid muscle *(cut)*
Digastric muscle (anterior belly)
Submandibular gland
Facial artery and vein
Hyoid bone
Parotid gland
Retromandibular vein (anterior and posterior branches)
Digastric muscle (posterior belly)
Stylohyoid muscle
External jugular vein
Sternocleidomastoid muscle
Common trunk receiving facial, anterior branch of retromandibular, and lingual veins (common facial vein)
Internal jugular vein
External carotid artery

Parotid gland: totally serous

Submandibular gland: mostly serous, partially mucous

Sublingual gland: almost completely mucous

Figure 3-12. The salivary glands.

Teeth (Figures 3-13 and 3-14 [p. 130])

The teeth develop and emerge from alveolar bone in the mandible and maxilla. The alveoli are covered externally by the gingivae or gums, which are made of fibrous conjunctive tissue. A normal adult has 32 permanent teeth, which are as follows (see Figure 3-14, p. 130):

- 8 incisors
- 4 canines, or cuspids
- 8 premolars, or bicuspids
- 12 molars, including the third molars, commonly called *wisdom teeth*
  Each tooth is composed of the following:
- The crown is the portion of the tooth that extends above the alveolar boundary.
- The root is the portion of the tooth attached to the alveolar bone of the maxilla or mandible. The dental hole, or canal, located at the extremity of the roots, allows for the dental nerves and the vessels.
- The cusp is the prominence on the occlusal surface of the tooth. Canines have one such prominence. Premolars have two, and molars have four or five.

  Surfaces are used to describe the external appearance of a tooth, and each tooth contains five surfaces, as follows:

1. Occlusal surface is the part of the tooth that is in contact with the tooth of the opposite jaw (maxilla or mandible).
2. Lingual surface is adjacent to the tongue.
3. Buccal surface is adjacent to the cheek for premolars and molars.
4. Labial surface is adjacent to the lips for incisors and canines.
5. Distal and mesial surfaces represent the sides of each tooth that are adjacent to other teeth in the same jaw (maxilla or mandible). The mesial surface is oriented anteriorly, and the distal surface is located posteriorly.

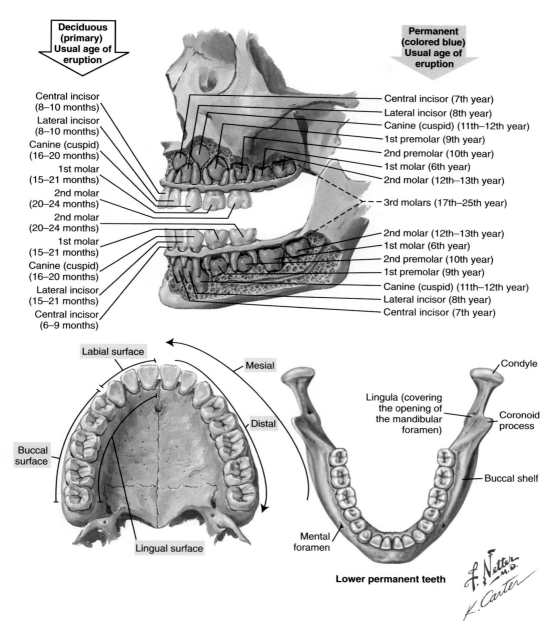

Deciduous (primary) Usual age of eruption

Central incisor (8–10 months)
Lateral incisor (8–10 months)
Canine (cuspid) (16–20 months)
1st molar (15–21 months)
2nd molar (20–24 months)

2nd molar (20–24 months)
1st molar (15–21 months)
Canine (cuspid) (16–20 months)
Lateral incisor (15–21 months)
Central incisor (6–9 months)

Permanent (colored blue) Usual age of eruption

Central incisor (7th year)
Lateral incisor (8th year)
Canine (cuspid) (11th–12th year)
1st premolar (9th year)
2nd premolar (10th year)
1st molar (6th year)
2nd molar (12th–13th year)

3rd molars (17th–25th year)

2nd molar (12th–13th year)
1st molar (6th year)
2nd premolar (10th year)
1st premolar (9th year)
Canine (cuspid) (11th–12th year)
Lateral incisor (8th year)
Central incisor (7th year)

Labial surface
Mesial
Distal
Buccal surface
Lingual surface

Condyle
Lingula (covering the opening of the mandibular foramen)
Coronoid process
Buccal shelf
Mental foramen

Lower permanent teeth

Figure 3-13. Teeth: age of eruption and surfaces.

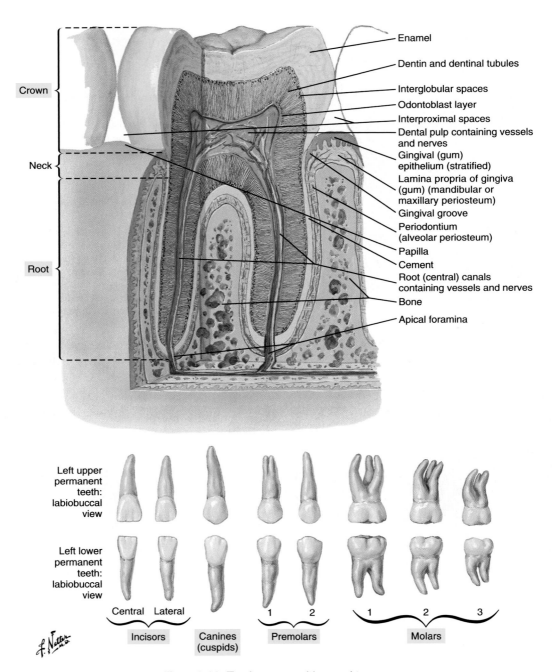

Crown

Neck

Root

Enamel

Dentin and dentinal tubules

Interglobular spaces

Odontoblast layer

Interproximal spaces

Dental pulp containing vessels and nerves

Gingival (gum) epithelium (stratified)

Lamina propria of gingiva (gum) (mandibular or maxillary periosteum)

Gingival groove

Periodontium (alveolar periosteum)

Papilla

Cement

Root (central) canals containing vessels and nerves

Bone

Apical foramina

Left upper permanent teeth: labiobuccal view

Left lower permanent teeth: labiobuccal view

Central   Lateral   1   2   1   2   3

Incisors   Canines   Premolars   Molars
(cuspids)

Figure 3-14. Teeth: composition and types.

Dental Occlusion

Globally, dental occlusion is the alignment and relationship between the teeth. Occlusion can also be defined as the normal contact between the occlusal surfaces of the teeth of the mandible and maxilla. The classification system of Dr. Edward H. Angle is often used, although not without controversy, to describe occlusal relationships between teeth. This system uses the relationship between the first molars of the mandible and maxilla and does not describe other potential problems with tooth alignment (e.g., crowding). Angle's system includes the following classifications:

- Class I neutral occlusion occurs when the first maxillary molar is slightly posterior and external to the first mandibular molar. More precisely, the mesiobuccal cusp of the first maxillary molar is aligned with the mesiobuccal groove (the one that separates the distal and mesial cusps) of the first mandibular molar.
- Class I malocclusion occurs when there is a neutral relationship between the molars, but there are problems with the alignment of anterior (mesial) teeth.
- Class II ("overbite") occurs when the first maxillary molar is anterior to the first mandibular molar or aligned with the first mandibular molar. More precisely, the mesiobuccal cusp of the first maxillary molar is anterior to the mesiobuccal cusp (the one that separates the distal and mesial cusps) of the first mandibular molar. Class II is divided into the following:
  - Division I, in which the relationship between the central incisors is normal (i.e., the maxillary central incisors are in protrusion and slightly overhang the mandibular central incisors).
  - Division II, in which the relationship between the central incisors is abnormal (i.e., the maxillary central incisors, even if they are anterior to the mandibular incisors, are in retraction and inclined toward the tongue).
- Class III ("underbite") occurs when the first maxillary molar is significantly posterior to the first mandibular molar. More precisely, the mesiobuccal cusp of the first maxillary molar is posterior to the mesiobuccal groove (the one that separates the distal and mesial cusps) of the first mandibular molar.

■ MUSCLES OF THE LIPS AND FACIAL EXPRESSION
(Figure 3-15; see Figure 3-16, p. 135)

The muscles of the lips and facial expression are not always attached from bone to bone or bone to cartilage. Rather, many originate from a bone and insert on the skin or on other muscles. A complex orientation and interdigitation of lip muscle fibers underlie the synergistic actions of these muscles to generate the precise movements necessary for facial expression, social interaction, speech production, mastication, and swallowing. The considerable complexity of facial and lip musculature combined with variability in location and morphology across individuals (which may be due to differences in facial size and shape) make exact determinations of muscle function difficult.

We will concentrate on muscles of the midface, lower face, and neck, and muscles will be classified in relationship to the orbicularis oris muscle, giving rise to transverse, angular, and vertical muscles.

Orbicularis Oris Muscle

The orbicularis oris muscle is composed of primarily horizontally oriented muscle fibers that encircle the mouth in four quadrants: left, right, superior, and inferior, with each quadrant fanning out from the modiolus to the facial midline. Muscle fibers in each quadrant can be further delineated into marginal portions (pars marginalis), deep to the vermilion, and peripheral portions (pars peripheralis), around the lips.

Once thought to have a simple sphincter-like or constrictor function, our current understanding is of a much more complex muscle whose actions depend on the co-activation of other facial muscles. The orbicularis oris muscle is involved in lip compression for mastication, swallowing, and speech sound production.

The orbicularis oris muscle is innervated by the buccal branches of the facial nerve (cranial nerve VII).

Two Transverse Muscles

Buccinator Muscle (see Figure 3-15)
The buccinator muscle is a deep facial muscle and a primary muscle of the cheeks. To obtain a good view of this muscle, we have to remove the masseter, which is an important jaw-closing muscle. The buccinator is a quadrilateral muscle that originates from the pterygomandibular raphe (ligament) and the molar alveolar processes of the mandible and maxilla. Muscle fibers course anteriorly (horizontally) to insert into the modiolus and the superior and inferior portions of the orbicularis oris muscle (crossed and uncrossed fibers) at the angle of the mouth. Muscle contraction pulls the lips laterally (retraction), compresses the cheeks, and assists in manipulating the food bolus during mastication and swallowing.

The buccinator muscle is innervated by the buccal branch of the facial nerve (cranial nerve VII).

Risorius Muscle (see Figure 3-16, p. 135)
The risorius muscle shows considerable individual variability and is often absent. It is parallel and superficial to the buccinator muscle. It originates from the fascia above the parotid gland and the aponeurosis of the masseter muscle and inserts into the modiolus. Muscular contraction pulls the lips laterally, as in smiling.

The risorius is innervated by the zygomatic and buccal branches of the facial nerve (cranial nerve VII).

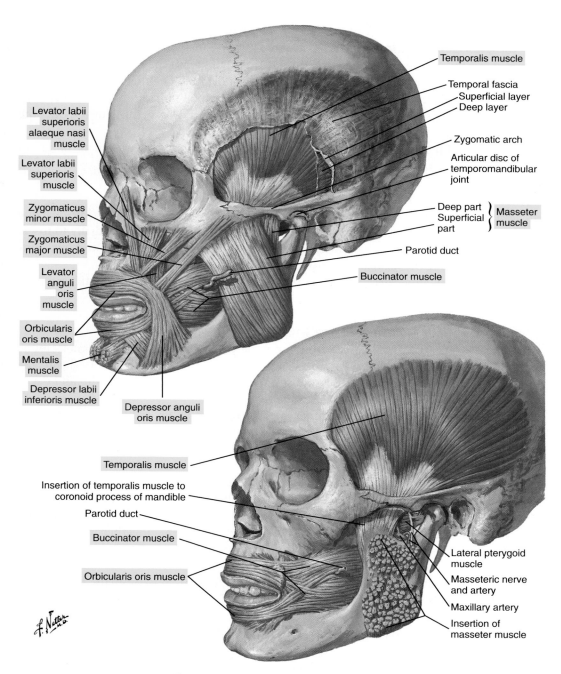

Temporalis muscle

Temporal fascia
Superficial layer
Deep layer

Zygomatic arch

Articular disc of
temporomandibular
joint

Deep part
Superficial
part
} Masseter
muscle

Parotid duct

Buccinator muscle

Levator labii
superioris
alaeque nasi
muscle

Levator labii
superioris
muscle

Zygomaticus
minor muscle

Zygomaticus
major muscle

Levator
anguli
oris
muscle

Orbicularis
oris muscle

Mentalis
muscle

Depressor labii
inferioris muscle

Depressor anguli
oris muscle

Temporalis muscle

Insertion of temporalis muscle to
coronoid process of mandible

Parotid duct

Buccinator muscle

Orbicularis oris muscle

Lateral pterygoid
muscle

Masseteric nerve
and artery

Maxillary artery

Insertion of
masseter muscle

Figure 3-15. The muscles of mastication.

Five Angular Muscles

Levator Labii Superioris Alaeque Nasi Muscle (Figure 3-16)

The levator labii superioris alaeque nasi muscle originates from the frontal process of the maxilla and divides into medial and lateral muscular portions. The medial portion inserts into the alar cartilage and acts to dilate the nostril. The lateral portion inserts into the lateral portion of the superior orbicularis muscle, elevates and everts (turns inside out) the upper lip, and may deepen the nasolabial sulcus.

The levator labii superioris alaeque nasi muscle is innervated by the zygomatic and buccal branches of the facial nerve (cranial nerve VII).

Levator Labii Superioris Muscle (see Figure 3-16)

The levator labii superioris muscle originates lateral to the levator labii superioris alaeque nasi muscle from the inferior surface of the orbit to head inferiorly and medially to insert into the superior orbicularis oris muscle. It elevates and everts the upper lip and may contribute to deepening the nasolabial furrow.

The levator labii superioris (superior) muscle is innervated by the zygomatic and buccal branches of the facial nerve (cranial nerve VII).

Zygomaticus Minor Muscle (see Figure 3-16)

Sometimes absent, the zygomaticus minor muscle originates from the zygomatic bone lateral to the levator labii superioris and heads inferiorly and medially to insert into the superior portion of the orbicularis oris muscle. Its action elevates the upper lip and deepens the nasolabial fold as in smiling.

The zygomaticus minor muscle is innervated by the zygomatic and buccal branches of the facial nerve (cranial nerve VII).

Zygomaticus Major Muscle (see Figure 3-16)

The zygomaticus major muscle originates from the zygomatic bone, lateral to the zygomaticus minor muscle. It heads inferiorly and medially to insert into the superior portion of the orbicularis oris muscle and the modiolus. It is often composed of superficial and deep portions, with the levator anguli oris passing between them. Together with the levator anguli oris, its action pulls the lips superiorly and laterally such as when smiling or laughing.

The zygomaticus major muscle is innervated by the buccal and zygomatic branches of the facial nerve (cranial nerve VII).

Depressor Labii Inferioris Muscle (see Figures 3-15 [p. 133] and 3-16)

The depressor labii inferioris muscle originates from the external oblique line of the mandible. It heads superiorly and medially to insert into the modiolus and the inferior orbicularis oris muscle. Its action pulls the lower lip down during mastication and may contribute to facial expressions such as sadness or sorrow.

The depressor labii inferioris muscle is innervated by the mandibular branch of the facial nerve (cranial nerve VII).

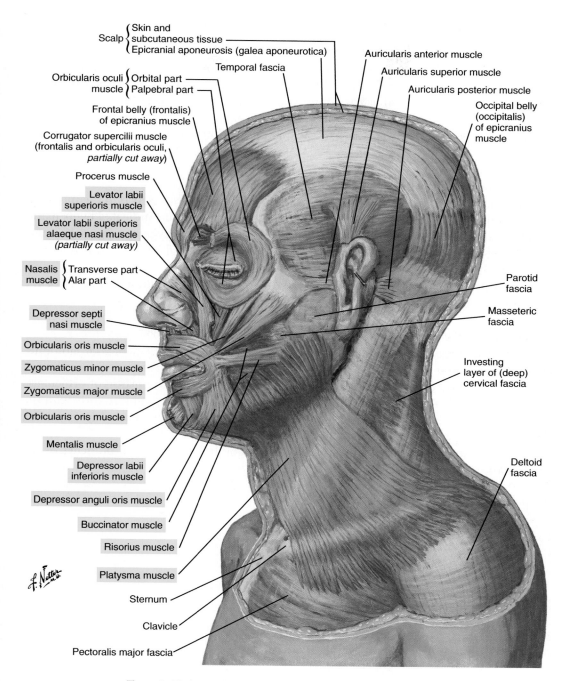

Scalp {
Skin and
subcutaneous tissue
Epicranial aponeurosis (galea aponeurotica)

Temporal fascia

Orbicularis oculi { Orbital part
muscle } Palpebral part

Frontal belly (frontalis)
of epicranius muscle

Corrugator supercilii muscle
(frontalis and orbicularis oculi,
partially cut away)

Procerus muscle

Levator labii
superioris muscle

Levator labii superioris
alaeque nasi muscle
(partially cut away)

Nasalis } Transverse part
muscle } Alar part

Depressor septi
nasi muscle

Orbicularis oris muscle

Zygomaticus minor muscle

Zygomaticus major muscle

Orbicularis oris muscle

Mentalis muscle

Depressor labii
inferioris muscle

Depressor anguli oris muscle

Buccinator muscle

Risorius muscle

Platysma muscle

Sternum

Clavicle

Pectoralis major fascia

Auricularis anterior muscle

Auricularis superior muscle

Auricularis posterior muscle

Occipital belly
(occipitalis)
of epicranius
muscle

Parotid
fascia

Masseteric
fascia

Investing
layer of (deep)
cervical fascia

Deltoid
fascia

Figure 3-16. Lateral view of the muscles of facial expression.

Three Vertical Muscles

Mentalis Muscle (see Figures 3-15 [p. 133] and 3-16 [p. 135])

The mentalis muscle originates from the anterior surface of the body of the mandible to insert on the skin of the chin and on the inferior portion of the orbicularis oris muscle and the modiolus. Its action elevates, protrudes, and everts the lower lip and may crease the chin.

The mentalis muscle is innervated by the mandibular branch of the facial nerve (cranial nerve VII).

Levator Anguli Oris Muscle (Caninus) (see Figure 3-15, p. 133)

The levator anguli oris muscle originates from the canine fossa to insert into the modiolus and the superior portion of the orbicularis oris superior muscle. As indicated by its name, its action elevates the angle of the mouth and, together with the zygomaticus major muscle, pulls the lips superiorly and laterally and deepens the nasolabial fold as in smiling or laughing.

The levator anguli oris muscle is innervated by zygomatic and buccal branches of the facial nerve (cranial nerve VII).

Depressor Anguli Oris Muscle (see Figures 3-15 [p. 133] and 3-16 [p. 135])

The depressor anguli oris muscle partially covers and is lateral to the depressor labii inferioris muscle and is superficial to platysma. It originates from the external oblique line of the mandible and heads superiorly to the modiolus and the inferior portion of orbicularis oris. Superiorly it is continuous with the levator anguli oris muscle and inferiorly with the platysma muscle. Its action depresses the angle of the mouth, as indicated by its name, such as in an expression of sadness.

The depressor anguli oris is innervated by the mandibular and buccal branches of the facial nerve (cranial nerve VII).

■ ONE MUSCLE OF THE NECK

Platysma Muscle (see Figure 3-16, p. 135)

The platysma muscle is very thin, flat, and large. It covers the majority of anterior and lateral surfaces of the neck. Its extension is very variable. It is deep to the depressor anguli oris muscle. In most individuals, it extends to the cheeks and the muscles of the mouth and the modiolus. However, for some, it can spread even farther up to the muscles surrounding the eyes. When this muscle contracts, it expands the neck and pulls the skin of the neck upward, which may also facilitate the drainage of nearby blood vessels. Also, this muscle may play a role in the downward movements of the lower lip and jaw.

The platysma is innervated by the cervical branch of the facial nerve (cranial nerve VII).

■ MUSCLES OF THE TONGUE (see Figure 3-11, p. 125)

At a functional level, the tongue can be divided into the following sections:
- The body constitutes the major mass of the tongue.
- The root is the posterior portion that forms the anterior boundary of the pharyngeal cavity.
- The dorsum is the dorsal surface of the tongue.
- The blade is the anterior part of the tongue, just behind the apex and beneath the alveolar ridge of the maxilla.
- The apex is the tip or the most anterior portion of the tongue.

These parts are particularly important for the tongue's actions for the production of the sounds of speech and for swallowing.

The tongue is composed of and controlled by the following two groups of muscles:
1. Intrinsic muscles have origins and insertions inside the tongue.
2. Extrinsic muscles have an origin outside the tongue and an insertion in the tongue.

Intrinsic Muscles of the Tongue (Figure 3-17)

The intrinsic muscles form a complex array of interdigitating muscle fibers. This complex arrangement allows for precise adjustments in tongue form and position. There are four intrinsic muscles, as follows:
1. Superior longitudinal muscle
2. Inferior longitudinal muscle
3. Transverse lingual muscle
4. Vertical lingual muscle

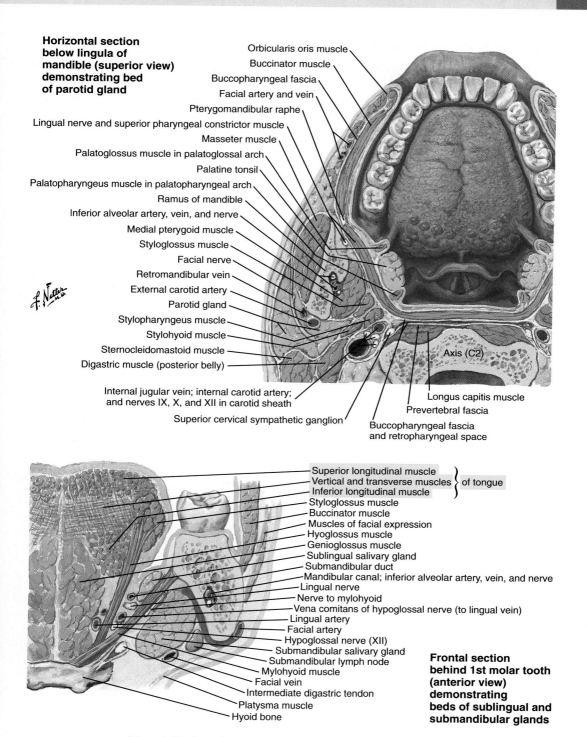

Horizontal section below lingula of mandible (superior view) demonstrating bed of parotid gland

Orbicularis oris muscle

Buccinator muscle

Buccopharyngeal fascia

Facial artery and vein

Pterygomandibular raphe

Lingual nerve and superior pharyngeal constrictor muscle

Masseter muscle

Palatoglossus muscle in palatoglossal arch

Palatine tonsil

Palatopharyngeus muscle in palatopharyngeal arch

Ramus of mandible

Inferior alveolar artery, vein, and nerve

Medial pterygoid muscle

Styloglossus muscle

Facial nerve

Retromandibular vein

External carotid artery

Parotid gland

Stylopharyngeus muscle

Stylohyoid muscle

Sternocleidomastoid muscle

Digastric muscle (posterior belly)

Internal jugular vein; internal carotid artery; and nerves IX, X, and XII in carotid sheath

Superior cervical sympathetic ganglion

Axis (C2)

Longus capitis muscle

Prevertebral fascia

Buccopharyngeal fascia and retropharyngeal space

Superior longitudinal muscle

Vertical and transverse muscles } of tongue

Inferior longitudinal muscle

Styloglossus muscle

Buccinator muscle

Muscles of facial expression

Hyoglossus muscle

Genioglossus muscle

Sublingual salivary gland

Submandibular duct

Mandibular canal; inferior alveolar artery, vein, and nerve

Lingual nerve

Nerve to mylohyoid

Vena comitans of hypoglossal nerve (to lingual vein)

Lingual artery

Facial artery

Hypoglossal nerve (XII)

Submandibular salivary gland

Submandibular lymph node

Mylohyoid muscle

Facial vein

Intermediate digastric tendon

Platysma muscle

Hyoid bone

Frontal section behind 1st molar tooth (anterior view) demonstrating beds of sublingual and submandibular glands

Figure 3-17. Superior view and coronal section of the tongue.

Extrinsic Muscles of the Tongue (Figure 3-18)

Extrinsic muscles link the tongue with surrounding structures. These muscles allow the tongue to move forward, backward, upward, downward, and laterally. Each name includes the word *glossus,* which means tongue, and another term indicating the external origin. There are four extrinsic muscles, as follows:

1. Palatoglossus muscle
2. Styloglossus muscle
3. Hyoglossus muscle
4. Genioglossus muscle

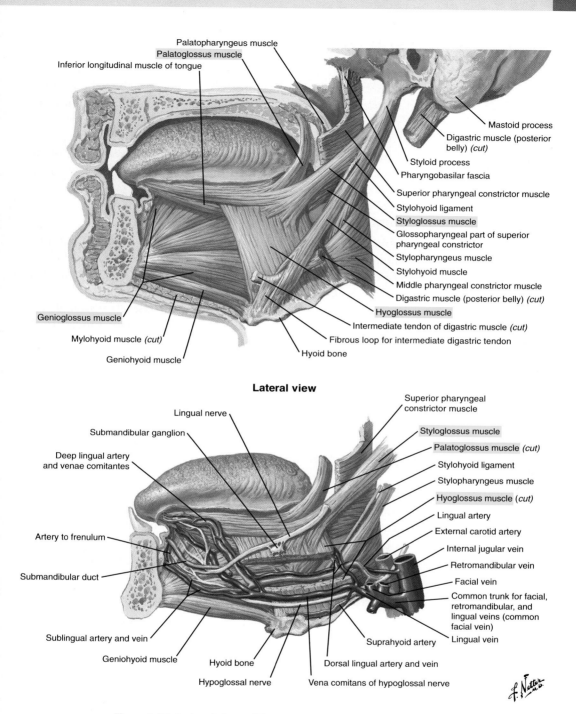

Palatopharyngeus muscle
Palatoglossus muscle
Inferior longitudinal muscle of tongue

Mastoid process
Digastric muscle (posterior belly) *(cut)*
Styloid process
Pharyngobasilar fascia
Superior pharyngeal constrictor muscle
Stylohyoid ligament
Styloglossus muscle
Glossopharyngeal part of superior pharyngeal constrictor
Stylopharyngeus muscle
Stylohyoid muscle
Middle pharyngeal constrictor muscle
Digastric muscle (posterior belly) *(cut)*
Hyoglossus muscle
Intermediate tendon of digastric muscle *(cut)*
Fibrous loop for intermediate digastric tendon
Hyoid bone

Genioglossus muscle
Mylohyoid muscle *(cut)*
Geniohyoid muscle

Lateral view

Lingual nerve
Submandibular ganglion
Deep lingual artery and venae comitantes

Superior pharyngeal constrictor muscle
Styloglossus muscle
Palatoglossus muscle *(cut)*
Stylohyoid ligament
Stylopharyngeus muscle
Hyoglossus muscle *(cut)*
Lingual artery
External carotid artery
Internal jugular vein
Retromandibular vein
Facial vein
Common trunk for facial, retromandibular, and lingual veins (common facial vein)
Lingual vein

Artery to frenulum
Submandibular duct

Sublingual artery and vein
Geniohyoid muscle
Hyoid bone
Hypoglossal nerve
Suprahyoid artery
Dorsal lingual artery and vein
Vena comitans of hypoglossal nerve

Figure 3-18. Lateral view of the tongue and associated muscles.

◼ MUSCLES OF MASTICATION

Mastication is the process of food reduction and preparation for swallowing. It requires the complex coordinated movements of the jaw, lips, cheeks, and tongue. The origin of jaw muscles, often called *muscles of mastication*, is typically on the skull and the insertion of jaw muscles is on the mandible, which is the movable portion of the jaw around the temporomandibular joint. Clearly, movements of the jaw are important for speech production, and as a result of biomechanical linkage, they influence the lips and the tongue. The muscles of mastication can generally be divided into jaw-opening and jaw-closing muscles, or jaw elevators and jaw depressors, respectively.

Temporomandibular Joint (Figure 3-19)

The temporomandibular joint is a synovial joint between the condyle of the mandible and the mandibular (articular, glenoid) fossa of the temporal bone. The articular surfaces of both structures are covered with fibrocartilage and separated by and connected to a cartilaginous articular disc. An articular capsule (articular ligament) surrounds these structures and thickens laterally to form the temporomandibular (lateral) ligament. This ligament courses from the mandible to the articular tubercle and zygomatic process of the temporal bone. Two other ligaments, the stylomandibular ligament and the sphenomandibular ligament, both located medially, may provide some additional support.

Two movements are associated with the temporomandibular joint, as follows:

1. Translation is a gliding type of movement that can be either bilateral (backward-forward movements of the jaw) or unilateral (the mandible moves from one side to the other).
2. Rotation is a "hinge"-type movement of the jaw. Imagine the jaw rotating around an imaginary horizontal axis through the condylar processes of the two sides of the mandible.

Mastication and speech involve a combination of these two types of jaw movements, with specific movement trajectories influenced by the nature of the food bolus and the position within the masticatory sequence (from food ingestion to swallowing for mastication) and the specific speech sound produced and phonetic environment (for speech). There is also individual variability in both masticatory and speech movements.

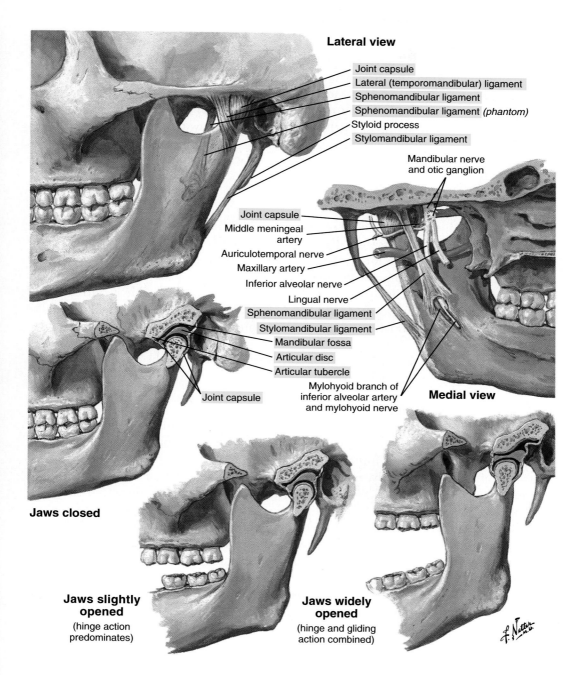

Lateral view

Joint capsule
Lateral (temporomandibular) ligament
Sphenomandibular ligament
Sphenomandibular ligament *(phantom)*
Styloid process
Stylomandibular ligament

Mandibular nerve
and otic ganglion

Joint capsule
Middle meningeal
artery
Auriculotemporal nerve
Maxillary artery
Inferior alveolar nerve
Lingual nerve
Sphenomandibular ligament
Stylomandibular ligament
Mandibular fossa
Articular disc
Articular tubercle
Joint capsule

Mylohyoid branch of
inferior alveolar artery
and mylohyoid nerve

Medial view

Jaws closed

**Jaws slightly
opened**
(hinge action
predominates)

**Jaws widely
opened**
(hinge and gliding
action combined)

Figure 3-19. The temporomandibular joint.

Three Jaw Closing Muscles (Jaw Elevators)

Masseter Muscle (see Figure 3-15, p. 133)

The masseter muscle has superficial (external) and deep (internal) fibers. The masseter muscle originates from the zygomatic process of the maxilla and the zygomatic arch. Fibers travel inferiorly to insert on the external surface of the angle and ramus of the mandible. Some fibers also insert on the coronoid process of the mandible. The masseter elevates the mandible. Superficial fibers may contribute to jaw protrusion and deep fibers to jaw retraction.

The masseter muscle is innervated by the mandibular branch of the trigeminal nerve (cranial nerve V).

Temporalis Muscle (see Figure 3-15, p. 133)

The temporalis muscle is composed of anterior, middle, and posterior portions. It originates from the temporal fossa on the parietal and temporal bones. Its fibers converge under the zygomatic arch to form a tendon that inserts on the coronoid process and the anterior surface of the ramus of the mandible. Contraction of the anterior and middle portions, composed principally of vertical fibers, elevates the mandible. Contraction of the posterior portion, which is made of more horizontal fibers, may elevate and retract the mandible. Unilateral contraction of these muscle fibers may contribute to lateral movements of the jaw.

The temporalis muscle is innervated by the temporal nerve of the mandibular branch of the trigeminal nerve (cranial nerve V).

Medial (Internal) Pterygoid Muscle (Figure 3-20)

The medial (internal) pterygoid muscle originates primarily from the medial surface of the lateral pterygoid plate of the sphenoid bone. A small group of fibers originates from the maxillary tuberosity and from the perpendicular plate of the palatine bone. The fibers travel inferiorly, posteriorly, and laterally to insert on the internal surface of the angle and ramus of the mandible. This muscle forms, with the masseter muscle, a sling that surrounds the angle of the mandible and works with the masseter muscle and temporalis muscle to elevate the jaw. It acts in synergy with the lateral pterygoid muscle and the masseter muscle for jaw protrusion. Unilateral contraction of the medial pterygoid muscle moves the mandible laterally toward the opposite side. This action permits grinding movements during mastication.

The medial pterygoid muscle is innervated by the medial pterygoid nerve of the mandibular branch of the trigeminal nerve (cranial nerve V).

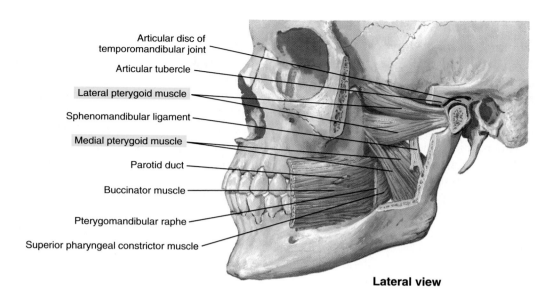

Articular disc of
temporomandibular joint

Articular tubercle

Lateral pterygoid muscle

Sphenomandibular ligament

Medial pterygoid muscle

Parotid duct

Buccinator muscle

Pterygomandibular raphe

Superior pharyngeal constrictor muscle

Lateral view

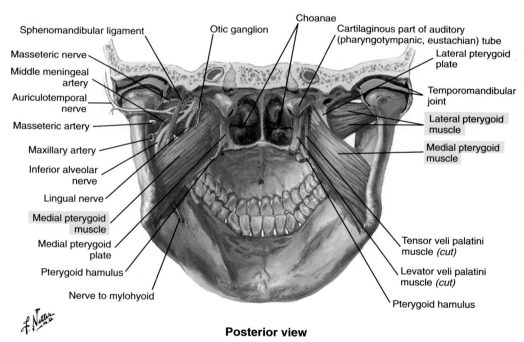

Sphenomandibular ligament

Masseteric nerve

Middle meningeal artery

Auriculotemporal nerve

Masseteric artery

Maxillary artery

Inferior alveolar nerve

Lingual nerve

Medial pterygoid muscle

Medial pterygoid plate

Pterygoid hamulus

Nerve to mylohyoid

Otic ganglion

Choanae

Cartilaginous part of auditory (pharyngotympanic, eustachian) tube

Lateral pterygoid plate

Temporomandibular joint

Lateral pterygoid muscle

Medial pterygoid muscle

Tensor veli palatini muscle *(cut)*

Levator veli palatini muscle *(cut)*

Pterygoid hamulus

Posterior view

Figure 3-20. Lateral and posterior views of the muscles of mastication.

Four Jaw Opening Muscles (Jaw Depressors)

Lateral (External) Pterygoid Muscle (see Figure 3-20, p. 145)

The lateral (external) pterygoid muscle has two heads. The superior portion originates from the fossa of the greater wing of the sphenoid bone and the inferior portion from the external surface of the lateral pterygoid plate of the sphenoid bone. Fibers course horizontally to insert on the articular disc of the temporomandibular joint and on the condyle of the mandible. The superior portion of this muscle is co-activated with jaw-closing muscles during mastication. The bilateral contraction of the inferior portion protrudes the mandible. The alternating unilateral contraction of the inferior portion produces a lateral movement of the mandible toward the opposite side.

The lateral pterygoid muscle is innervated by the mandibular branch nerve of the trigeminal nerve (cranial nerve V).

Digastric Muscle (Figures 3-21 and 3-22, pp. 148-149)

The digastric muscle is frequently classified as a suprahyoid muscle. This muscle contains posterior and anterior "bellies" (hence its name) that are linked by a central tendon. This central tendon is fixed to the hyoid bone by a loop-shaped intermediate tendon.

The posterior belly originates from the mastoid process of the temporal bone. Muscular contraction contributes to the elevation of the hyoid bone. The anterior belly originates from the internal surface of the inferior border of the mandible and travels posteriorly to insert on the hyoid bone. With the hyoid bone fixed by other muscles, the anterior belly of the digastric muscle acts as a jaw opener.

The posterior belly of the digastric muscle is innervated by the digastric branch of the facial nerve (cranial nerve VII), and the anterior belly of the digastric muscle is innervated by the mylohyoid branch of the inferior alveolar nerve of the mandibular branch of the trigeminal nerve (cranial nerve V).

Mylohyoid Muscle (see Figures 3-21 and 3-22, pp. 148-149)

The mylohyoid muscle originates from the mylohyoid line (internal oblique line) of the mandible. The anterior and middle fibers insert into the median mylohyoid raphe joined by muscular fibers of the opposite side. The posterior fibers insert on the hyoid bone. The mylohyoid is fan-shaped and contributes to the muscular floor of the mouth. Contraction elevates the floor of the mouth, the hyoid, and the tongue. It can also contribute to jaw opening if the hyoid bone is fixed.

The mylohyoid muscle is innervated by the mylohyoid branch of the inferior alveolar nerve of the mandibular branch of the trigeminal nerve (cranial nerve V).

Geniohyoid Muscle (see Figure 3-22, p. 149)

The geniohyoid muscle extends from the internal surface of the mandibular symphysis to the hyoid bone. Two bellies are located on each side of the median line and almost parallel to the anterior bellies of the digastric muscle, which are inferior. Contraction of the mylohyoid and the geniohyoid muscles may retract the jaw. Their contraction also contributes to jaw opening if the anterior belly of the digastric muscle is activated and the hyoid bone is stabilized.

The geniohyoid muscle is innervated by the first cervical spinal nerve (C1) traveling with the fibers of the hypoglossal nerve (cranial nerve XII).

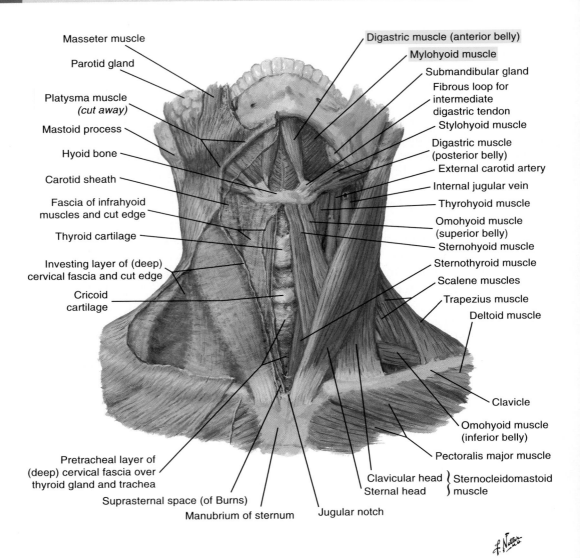

Masseter muscle

Parotid gland

Platysma muscle
(cut away)

Mastoid process

Hyoid bone

Carotid sheath

Fascia of infrahyoid
muscles and cut edge

Thyroid cartilage

Investing layer of (deep)
cervical fascia and cut edge

Cricoid
cartilage

Digastric muscle (anterior belly)

Mylohyoid muscle

Submandibular gland

Fibrous loop for
intermediate
digastric tendon

Stylohyoid muscle

Digastric muscle
(posterior belly)

External carotid artery

Internal jugular vein

Thyrohyoid muscle

Omohyoid muscle
(superior belly)

Sternohyoid muscle

Sternothyroid muscle

Scalene muscles

Trapezius muscle

Deltoid muscle

Clavicle

Omohyoid muscle
(inferior belly)

Pectoralis major muscle

Clavicular head ⎫ Sternocleidomastoid
Sternal head   ⎬ muscle

Pretracheal layer of
(deep) cervical fascia over
thyroid gland and trachea

Suprasternal space (of Burns)

Manubrium of sternum

Jugular notch

Figure 3-21. Anterior view of the neck. Note the anterior belly of the digastric and the mylohyoid muscles, both jaw openers.

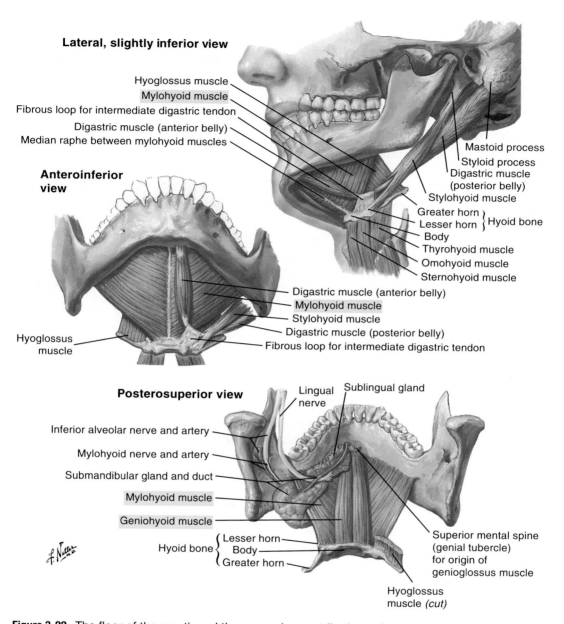

Lateral, slightly inferior view

Hyoglossus muscle
Mylohyoid muscle
Fibrous loop for intermediate digastric tendon
Digastric muscle (anterior belly)
Median raphe between mylohyoid muscles

Mastoid process
Styloid process
Digastric muscle (posterior belly)
Stylohyoid muscle
Greater horn
Lesser horn } Hyoid bone
Body
Thyrohyoid muscle
Omohyoid muscle
Sternohyoid muscle

Anteroinferior view

Digastric muscle (anterior belly)
Mylohyoid muscle
Stylohyoid muscle
Digastric muscle (posterior belly)
Fibrous loop for intermediate digastric tendon

Hyoglossus muscle

Posterosuperior view

Lingual nerve
Sublingual gland

Inferior alveolar nerve and artery
Mylohyoid nerve and artery
Submandibular gland and duct
Mylohyoid muscle
Geniohyoid muscle

Hyoid bone { Lesser horn
Body
Greater horn

Superior mental spine (genial tubercle) for origin of genioglossus muscle

Hyoglossus muscle (cut)

Figure 3-22. The floor of the mouth and three muscles contributing to jaw opening: (1) the anterior belly of the digastric, (2) the mylohyoid, and (3) the geniohyoid.

■ MUSCLES OF THE SOFT PALATE (Figure 3-23)

The soft palate, or velum, is a posterior extension of the hard or bony palate. It is formed principally by five muscles: the levator veli palatini, the tensor veli palatini, the palatoglossus, the palatopharyngeus, and the uvular. The only intrinsic muscle of the soft palate is the uvular muscle. All other muscles have an exterior attachment.

Levator Veli Palatini Muscle (see Figure 3-23)

The levator veli palatini muscle is a palatal elevator. Fibers originate from the petrous portion of the temporal bone and the inferior aspect of the cartilaginous auditory (pharyngotympanic, eustachian) tube. Fibers travel inferiorly and toward the midline to insert into the palatine raphe (aponeurosis) of the soft palate. Contraction of this muscle pulls the soft palate toward the posterior pharyngeal wall. The role of this muscle in contributing to the opening of the eustachian tube (auditory tube) for the ventilation of the middle ear is controversial (see Figure 3-9, p. 121).

The levator veli palatini muscle is innervated by the spinal accessory nerve (cranial nerve XI) via the pharyngeal branch of the vagus nerve (cranial nerve X) and the pharyngeal plexus.

Tensor Veli Palatini Muscle (see Figure 3-23; see also Figure 3-8, p. 119)

The tensor veli palatini muscle has three origins: the medial pterygoid plate and scaphoid fossa, the spine of the sphenoid bone, and the lateral cartilaginous walls of the eustachian tube. The fibers from the superior origin go forward and downward to join the tendon surrounding the hamulus and insert into the palatine raphe (aponeurosis). This muscle dilates the eustachian tube and may also tense the palate.

The tensor veli palatini muscle is innervated by the mandibular branch of the trigeminal nerve (cranial nerve V).

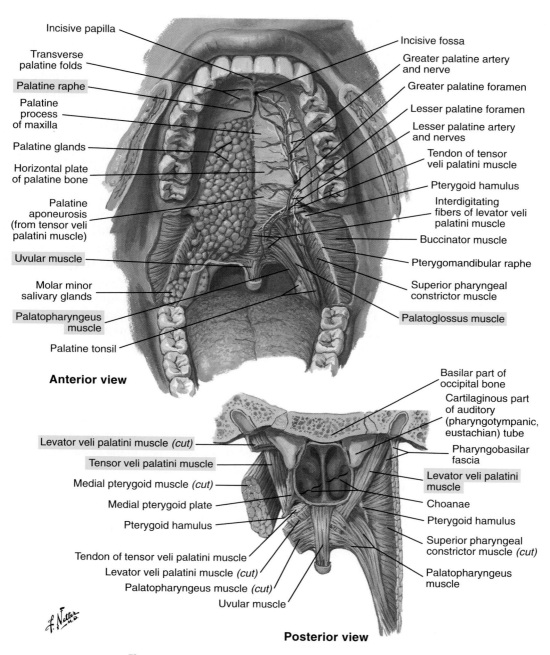

Anterior view

- Incisive papilla
- Transverse palatine folds
- Palatine raphe
- Palatine process of maxilla
- Palatine glands
- Horizontal plate of palatine bone
- Palatine aponeurosis (from tensor veli palatini muscle)
- Uvular muscle
- Molar minor salivary glands
- Palatopharyngeus muscle
- Palatine tonsil

- Incisive fossa
- Greater palatine artery and nerve
- Greater palatine foramen
- Lesser palatine foramen
- Lesser palatine artery and nerves
- Tendon of tensor veli palatini muscle
- Pterygoid hamulus
- Interdigitating fibers of levator veli palatini muscle
- Buccinator muscle
- Pterygomandibular raphe
- Superior pharyngeal constrictor muscle
- Palatoglossus muscle

Posterior view

- Levator veli palatini muscle *(cut)*
- Tensor veli palatini muscle
- Medial pterygoid muscle *(cut)*
- Medial pterygoid plate
- Pterygoid hamulus
- Tendon of tensor veli palatini muscle
- Levator veli palatini muscle *(cut)*
- Palatopharyngeus muscle *(cut)*
- Uvular muscle

- Basilar part of occipital bone
- Cartilaginous part of auditory (pharyngotympanic, eustachian) tube
- Pharyngobasilar fascia
- Levator veli palatini muscle
- Choanae
- Pterygoid hamulus
- Superior pharyngeal constrictor muscle *(cut)*
- Palatopharyngeus muscle

Figure 3-23. The soft palate and associated structures.

Palatoglossus (Glossopalatine) Muscle (see Figure 3-23, p. 151)

The palatoglossus (glossopalatine) muscle originates from the inferior surface of the palatine raphe (aponeurosis). Fibers course inferiorly to insert underneath the sides of the posterior portion of the tongue, principally on superficial muscles (located under the posterior portions of the sides of the tongue) and transverse muscles. The muscular fibers of the palatoglossus muscle form the bulk of the palatoglossal arch (or anterior faucial pillar) visible in the oral cavity. Contraction of this muscle may depress the soft palate or elevate the tongue with the soft palate fixed. This muscle approximates the palatoglossal arches.

The palatoglossus muscle is innervated by the spinal accessory nerve (cranial nerve XI) via the pharyngeal branch of the vagus nerve (cranial nerve X) and the pharyngeal plexus.

Palatopharyngeus Muscle (see Figure 3-23, p. 151)

The palatopharyngeus muscle originates from the palatine raphe (aponeurosis). Its fibers form the bulk of the palatopharyngeal arch (posterior faucial pillar). Fibers travel inferiorly with the muscular fibers of the stylopharyngeus muscle. The palatopharyngeus muscle inserts on the posterior border of the thyroid cartilage and on the inferior pharynx. Contraction of this muscle may depress the soft palate and elevate and constrict the pharynx and elevate the larynx. This muscle approximates the palatopharyngeal arches.

The palatopharyngeus muscle is innervated by the spinal accessory nerve (cranial nerve XI) via the pharyngeal branch of the vagus nerve (cranial nerve X) and the pharyngeal plexus.

Uvular Muscle (Musculus Uvulae) (see Figure 3-23, p. 151)

The uvular muscle extends from the posterior nasal spine and the palatine raphe (aponeurosis) to insert into the uvula. The function of this muscle is not well understood. However, it may play a role in the elevation of the soft palate. The uvula is an important landmark during an oral examination because its orientation and form may reflect anomalies of the hard and soft palate.

The uvular muscle is innervated by the spinal accessory nerve (cranial nerve XI) via the pharyngeal branch of the vagus nerve (cranial nerve X) and the pharyngeal plexus.

■ MUSCLES OF THE PHARYNX

Superior Pharyngeal Constrictor Muscle (Figure 3-24, p. 154)

The superior pharyngeal constrictor muscle forms a tube starting at the level of the ptery-gomandibular raphe. Its fibers circle around posteriorly to insert into the median pharyngeal raphe. This muscle forms the sides and the back of the nasopharynx and a part of the posterior wall of the oropharynx. Contraction of this muscle pulls the pharyngeal wall forward and reduces the pharyngeal diameter during swallowing, thus contributing to the contraction (or propulsive) pressure applied to the swallowed bolus. It also contributes to pharyngeal tone and plays a role in velopharyngeal closure, which is discussed in the next section.

The superior constrictor muscle is innervated by the spinal accessory nerve (cranial nerve XI) via the pharyngeal branch of the vagus nerve (cranial nerve X) and the pharyngeal plexus.

Middle Pharyngeal Constrictor Muscle (see Figure 3-24, p. 154)

The middle pharyngeal constrictor muscle originates from the greater horns of the hyoid bone and the stylohyoid ligament to circle posteriorly to insert in the median pharyngeal raphe. Its contraction reduces the diameter of the pharynx and contributes to the contraction (or propulsive) pressure applied to the swallowed bolus. It also contributes to pharyngeal tone.

The middle constrictor muscle is innervated by the spinal accessory nerve (cranial nerve XI) via the pharyngeal branch of the vagus nerve (cranial nerve X) and the pharyngeal plexus.

Inferior Pharyngeal Constrictor Muscle (see Figure 3-24, p. 154)

The inferior pharyngeal constrictor muscle exerts the most force of the pharyngeal constrictors. Some fibers originate from the sides of the cricoid cartilage to form the cricopharyngeus muscle, which forms the sphincter-like opening to the cervical esophagus during swallowing. A myotomized and residual form of this muscle and the pharynx are used to generate the esophageal sound source used by patients with laryngectomies. Swallowed air is expelled against a closed esophageal sphincter, causing it to vibrate.

Part of this muscle originates from the thyroid lamina and inserts on the median pharyngeal raphe. Contraction of this muscle reduces the diameter of the inferior part of the pharynx.

The inferior constrictor muscle is innervated by the spinal accessory nerve (cranial nerve XI) via the pharyngeal branch of the vagus nerve (cranial nerve X) and the pharyngeal plexus, as well as by the recurrent laryngeal nerve and external branch of the superior laryngeal nerve of the vagus nerve.

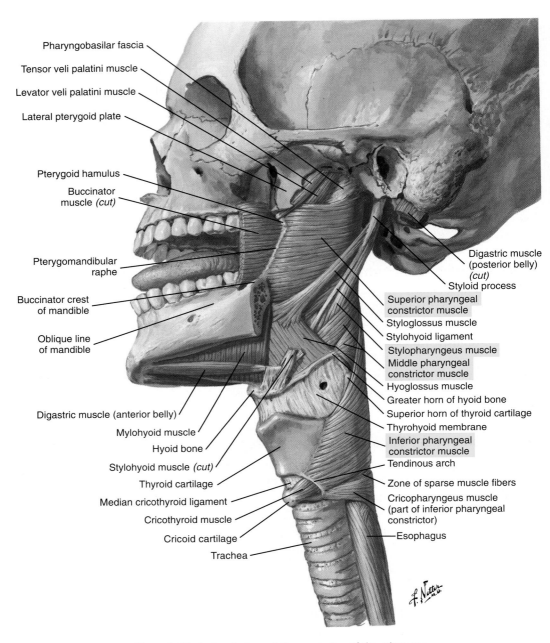

Pharyngobasilar fascia
Tensor veli palatini muscle
Levator veli palatini muscle
Lateral pterygoid plate

Pterygoid hamulus
Buccinator muscle *(cut)*

Pterygomandibular raphe

Buccinator crest of mandible

Oblique line of mandible

Digastric muscle (anterior belly)
Mylohyoid muscle
Hyoid bone
Stylohyoid muscle *(cut)*
Thyroid cartilage
Median cricothyroid ligament
Cricothyroid muscle
Cricoid cartilage
Trachea

Digastric muscle (posterior belly) *(cut)*
Styloid process
Superior pharyngeal constrictor muscle
Styloglossus muscle
Stylohyoid ligament
Stylopharyngeus muscle
Middle pharyngeal constrictor muscle
Hyoglossus muscle
Greater horn of hyoid bone
Superior horn of thyroid cartilage
Thyrohyoid membrane
Inferior pharyngeal constrictor muscle
Tendinous arch
Zone of sparse muscle fibers
Cricopharyngeus muscle (part of inferior pharyngeal constrictor)
Esophagus

Figure 3-24. Lateral view of the muscles of the pharynx.

Salpingopharyngeus Muscle (Figure 3-25, p. 156)

The salpingopharyngeus muscle originates at the inferoposterior surface of the cartilage of the eustachian tube and travels posteriorly to insert on the lateral walls of the pharynx. Its fibers mix with those of the palatopharyngeus muscle. Its contraction contributes to the elevation of the pharynx during swallowing and may contribute to the distortion of the tubal cartilage of the eustachian tube to permit aeration of the middle ear.

The salpingopharyngeus muscle is innervated by the spinal accessory nerve (cranial nerve XI) via the pharyngeal branch of the vagus nerve (cranial nerve X) and the pharyngeal plexus.

Stylopharyngeus Muscle (Figure 3-26, p. 157; see also Figure 3-24, p. 154)

The stylopharyngeus muscle constitutes a thin group of muscular fibers. Its origin is on the base of the styloid process of the temporal bone. It travels inferiorly and medially between the superior and middle pharyngeal constrictor muscles. This muscle inserts in the mucous membrane of the pharynx and on the thyroid cartilage. Its contraction elevates the larynx and elevates and expands the pharynx during swallowing.

The stylopharyngeus muscle is innervated by the glossopharyngeal nerve (cranial nerve IX).

Velopharyngeal Mechanism

The velopharyngeal mechanism (velopharyngeal closure) is an essential process for speech and swallowing. It involves the movement of many articulatory structures that act to modify the coupling between the nasal and oral cavities. Some speech sounds are produced with the laryngeal voice source passing only through the vocal tract, excluding the nasal cavities (oral sounds), and some are produced with both the oral and nasal cavities (nasal sounds). The velopharyngeal mechanism acts as a regulator for coupling or decoupling of the nasal cavity from the rest of the vocal tract. Elevating and retracting the soft palate and constricting the walls of the nasopharynx and anterior movements of the posterior wall of the pharynx blocks the nasal cavity for the production of oral sounds (p, d, g, b, t, k, and so on). Opposite movements of the velopharynx allow the laryngeal sound source to pass through and thus be modified by the nasal cavities. This creates the nasal sounds (m, n, and so on).

Velopharyngeal closure is an important airway protective mechanism for swallowing. Closure prevents food from entering the nasal passages during the passage of the bolus through the nasopharynx.

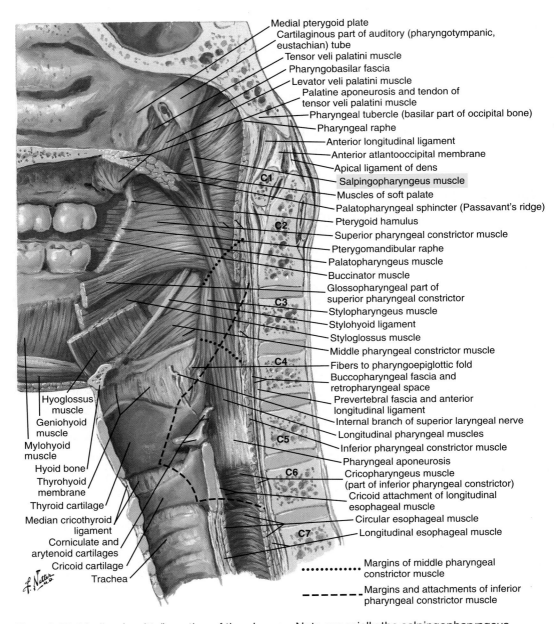

Medial pterygoid plate
Cartilaginous part of auditory (pharyngotympanic, eustachian) tube
Tensor veli palatini muscle
Pharyngobasilar fascia
Levator veli palatini muscle
Palatine aponeurosis and tendon of tensor veli palatini muscle
Pharyngeal tubercle (basilar part of occipital bone)
Pharyngeal raphe
Anterior longitudinal ligament
Anterior atlantooccipital membrane
Apical ligament of dens
Salpingopharyngeus muscle
Muscles of soft palate
Palatopharyngeal sphincter (Passavant's ridge)
Pterygoid hamulus
Superior pharyngeal constrictor muscle
Pterygomandibular raphe
Palatopharyngeus muscle
Buccinator muscle
Glossopharyngeal part of superior pharyngeal constrictor
Stylopharyngeus muscle
Stylohyoid ligament
Styloglossus muscle
Middle pharyngeal constrictor muscle
Fibers to pharyngoepiglottic fold
Buccopharyngeal fascia and retropharyngeal space
Prevertebral fascia and anterior longitudinal ligament
Internal branch of superior laryngeal nerve
Longitudinal pharyngeal muscles
Inferior pharyngeal constrictor muscle
Pharyngeal aponeurosis
Cricopharyngeus muscle (part of inferior pharyngeal constrictor)
Cricoid attachment of longitudinal esophageal muscle
Circular esophageal muscle
Longitudinal esophageal muscle

C1
C2
C3
C4
C5
C6
C7

Hyoglossus muscle
Geniohyoid muscle
Mylohyoid muscle
Hyoid bone
Thyrohyoid membrane
Thyroid cartilage
Median cricothyroid ligament
Corniculate and arytenoid cartilages
Cricoid cartilage
Trachea

•••••••••• Margins of middle pharyngeal constrictor muscle

– – – – – Margins and attachments of inferior pharyngeal constrictor muscle

Figure 3-25. Median (sagittal) section of the pharynx. Note especially the salpingopharyngeus muscle.

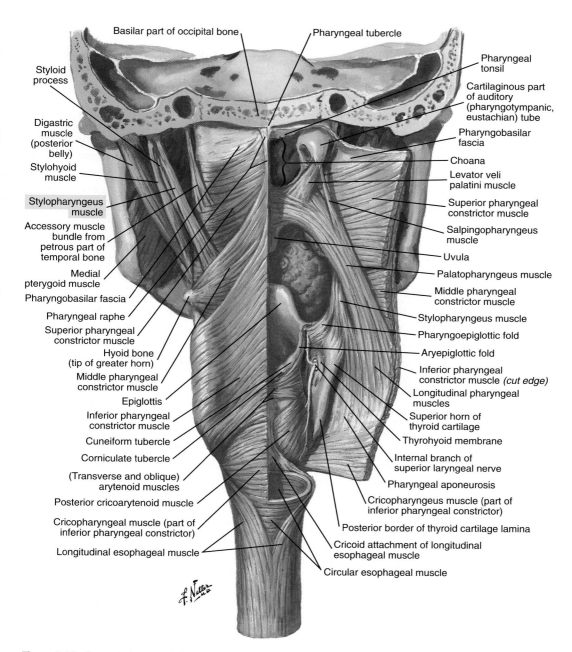

Figure 3-26. A posterior, partially reflected view of the pharynx. Note especially the stylopharyngeus muscle.

■ ESOPHAGUS (Figures 3-27, 3-28 [p. 160], and 3-29 [p. 161])

The esophagus is an important muscular tube that is involved in transporting solids and liquids from the pharynx to the stomach during swallowing. This complex structure is briefly summarized here.

Upper Esophageal, or Inferior Pharyngeal, Sphincter

The upper esophageal, or inferior pharyngeal, sphincter is the opening to the cervical esophagus from the pharynx. It is formed by the cricopharyngeus and inferior pharyngeal constrictor muscles. The sphincter is normally closed as a result of passive relaxation forces and tension provided by the cricopharyngeus and inferior pharyngeal constrictor and the apposition of the cricoid cartilage anteriorly. It opens by relaxation of the cricopharyngeus and inferior constrictor muscles and "actively" from laryngeal elevation by suprahyoid muscles (e.g., geniohyoid). The cricoid is "pulled away" from the posterior pharyngeal wall.

Primary Esophageal Peristalsis

Peristalsis is the process by which liquids or solids move through the esophagus by muscular contraction. It occurs subsequent to pharyngeal contraction and the opening of the upper esophageal sphincter. Contractions in striated (cervical) esophageal muscle (inner circular and outer longitudinal fibers) are followed by smooth (thoracic) muscular contractions. Secondary peristalsis may clear bolus residue.

Lower Esophageal Sphincter

The lower esophageal sphincter is the muscular junction between the esophagus and the stomach. It is closed to prevent gastroesophageal reflux by smooth esophageal muscle and crural portions of the diaphragm. The sphincter opens to accommodate the passage of the swallowed bolus into and out of the esophagus.

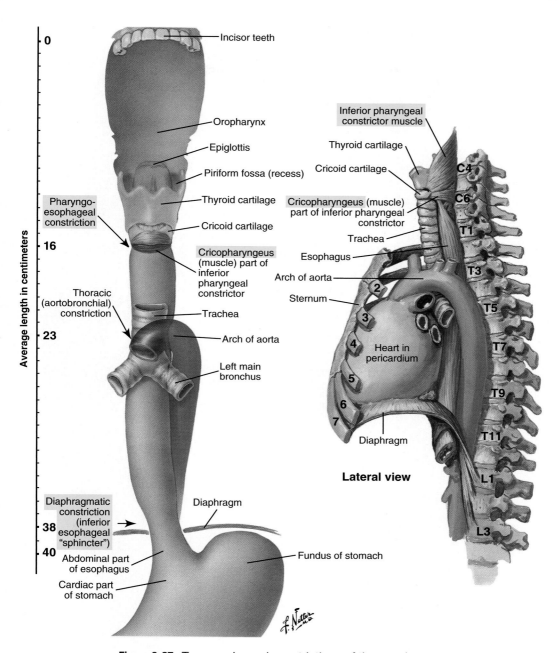

Figure 3-27. Topography and constrictions of the esophagus.

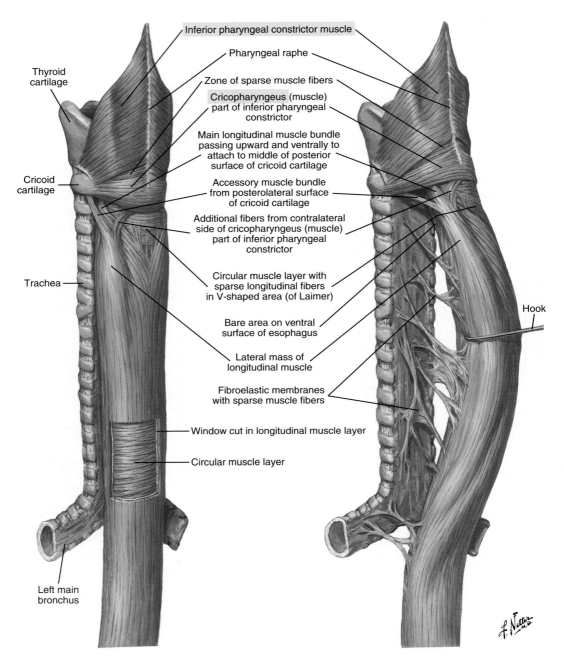

Figure 3-28. Musculature of the esophagus.

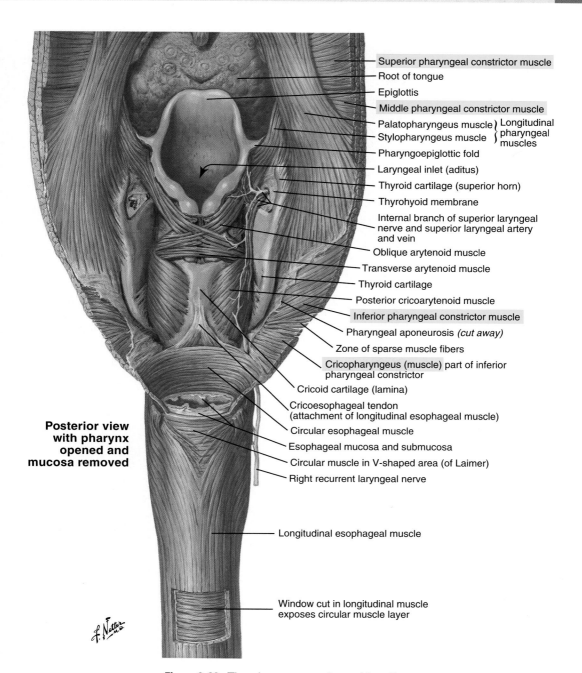

Superior pharyngeal constrictor muscle

Root of tongue

Epiglottis

Middle pharyngeal constrictor muscle

Palatopharyngeus muscle ⎱ Longitudinal
Stylopharyngeus muscle ⎰ pharyngeal
muscles

Pharyngoepiglottic fold

Laryngeal inlet (aditus)

Thyroid cartilage (superior horn)

Thyrohyoid membrane

Internal branch of superior laryngeal
nerve and superior laryngeal artery
and vein

Oblique arytenoid muscle

Transverse arytenoid muscle

Thyroid cartilage

Posterior cricoarytenoid muscle

Inferior pharyngeal constrictor muscle

Pharyngeal aponeurosis *(cut away)*

Zone of sparse muscle fibers

Cricopharyngeus (muscle) part of inferior
pharyngeal constrictor

Cricoid cartilage (lamina)

Cricoesophageal tendon
(attachment of longitudinal esophageal muscle)

Circular esophageal muscle

Esophageal mucosa and submucosa

Circular muscle in V-shaped area (of Laimer)

Right recurrent laryngeal nerve

**Posterior view
with pharynx
opened and
mucosa removed**

Longitudinal esophageal muscle

Window cut in longitudinal muscle
exposes circular muscle layer

Figure 3-29. The pharyngoesophageal junction.

Muscles of the Lips and Facial Expression (see Figures 3-15 [p. 133], and 3-16 [p. 135])

Muscle	Origin	Insertion	Action	Innervation
Muscles of the lips				
Orbicularis oris (pars marginalis and pars peripheralis)	Primarily horizontally oriented muscular fibers encircling the mouth from the modiolus	To the facial midline	Complex function depends on other co-activated muscles: • Closes the lips and projects them forward • Contracts and presses the lips against the incisors	Buccal branch of the facial nerve (cranial nerve VII)
Depressor anguli oris	External oblique line of the mandible	Modiolus and inferior portion of the orbicularis oris muscle	Depresses the angle of the mouth as in a sad expression	Mandibular and buccal branches of the facial nerve (cranial nerve VII)
Levator anguli oris	Canine fossa of the maxilla	Modiolus and superior portion of the orbicularis oris muscle	Pulls the corner of the lips superiorly and laterally and deepens the nasolabial fold as in smiling or laughing	Zygomatic and buccal branches of the facial nerve (cranial nerve VII)
Zygomaticus major	Zygomatic bone	Superior portion of the orbicularis oris muscle and modiolus	Pulls the lips superiorly and laterally, as when smiling or laughing	Buccal and zygomatic branches of the facial nerve (cranial nerve VII)
Risorius (variable muscle that is sometimes absent)	Fascia above the parotid gland Aponeurosis of the masseter muscle	Modiolus	Pulls the lips laterally, as in laughing	Zygomatic and buccal branches of the facial nerve (cranial nerve VII)
Levator labii superioris alaeque nasi	Frontal process of the maxilla	Medial portion: alar cartilage Lateral portion: superior orbicularis oris muscle	Medial portion: dilates nostril Lateral portion: elevates upper lip	Zygomatic and buccal branches of the facial nerve (cranial nerve VII)
Levator labii superioris	Inferior surface of the orbit	Superior orbicularis oris muscle	Elevates and everts the upper lip	Zygomatic and buccal branches of the facial nerve (cranial nerve VII)
Depressor labii inferioris	External oblique line of the mandible	Modiolus and inferior orbicularis oris muscle	Pulls the lower lip down and may contribute to expressions of sadness	Mandibular and buccal branches of the facial nerve (cranial nerve VII)

Zygomaticus minor (variable muscle that is sometimes absent)	Zygomatic bone	Superior portion of orbicularis oris muscle and modiolus	Elevates the upper lip and deepens the nasolabial fold, as in smiling	Zygomatic and buccal branches of the facial nerve (cranial nerve VII)
Muscle of the cheek				
Buccinator	Alveolar processes of the mandible and maxilla and pterygomandibular raphe (ligament), fibers course horizontally	Modiolus and superior orbicularis oris muscle and modiolus	Pulls the lips laterally Compresses the cheeks	Buccal branch of the facial nerve (cranial nerve VII)
Muscle of the chin				
Mentalis	Incisive fossa of the mandible	Skin of the chin Inferior orbicularis oris muscle	Elevates, protrudes, and everts the lower lip May crease the chin	Mandibular branch of the facial nerve (cranial nerve VII)
Muscles of the nose				
Nasalis Compressor naris	Maxilla	Bridge of the nose	Compresses the back of the nose	Zygomatic and buccal branches of the facial nerve (cranial nerve VII)
Nasalis Dilator naris	Nasal side of the maxillary bone	Alae of the nose	Dilates the nostrils	Zygomatic and buccal branches of the facial nerve (cranial nerve VII)
Depressor septi	Maxillary incisive fossa	Alae of the nose	Dilates the nostrils	Zygomatic and buccal branches of the facial nerve (cranial nerve VII)
Muscle of the neck				
Platysma	Fascia covering the deltoid muscle and the pectoralis muscle	Cheeks and muscles of the mouth and modiolus Some fibers may extend to muscles surrounding eyes (extent is variable)	Expands neck, pulls skin of neck upward, and depresses the lower lip and jaw	Cervical branch of the facial nerve (cranial nerve VII)

Muscles of the Tongue (see Figures 3-17 [p. 139], and 3-18 [p. 141])

Muscle	Origin	Insertion	Action	Innervation
Intrinsic tongue muscles				
Superior longitudinal	Fibrous tissue at the root and median fibrous septum	Fibrous membrane on the sides of the tongue	Shortens the tongue Turns the apex upward	Hypoglossal nerve (cranial nerve XII)
Inferior longitudinal	Root of the tongue	To the apex	Shortens the tongue Pulls the apex downward	Hypoglossal nerve (cranial nerve XII)
Transverse lingual	Median fibrous septum	Fibrous tissues at lateral margins	Makes the tongue narrower and elongates it	Hypoglossal nerve (cranial nerve XII)
Vertical lingual	Mucous membrane of tongue dorsum	Inferior and lateral tongue margins	Flattens and widens the tongue	Hypoglossal nerve (cranial nerve XII)
Extrinsic tongue muscles				
Palatoglossus	Inferior surface of palatal aponeurosis	Posterolateral portion of the tongue	Lifts the tongue Pulls it backward	Spinal accessory nerve (cranial nerve XI) via the pharyngeal plexus of the vagus nerve (cranial nerve X)
Styloglossus	Styloid process of the temporal bone Stylomandibular ligament	Posterolateral portion of the tongue	Lifts the sides of the tongue Pulls the tongue backward	Hypoglossal nerve (cranial nerve XII)
Hyoglossus	Greater horn and body of hyoid	Lateral sides of the tongue	Pulls down the sides of the tongue Pulls the tongue backward	Hypoglossal nerve (cranial nerve XII)
Genioglossus	Mental spine (genial tubercle) of the mandible	Back and apex of the tongue Inferior fibers insert on the hyoid bone	Protrudes the tongue and depresses central portion	Hypoglossal nerve (cranial nerve XII)

Muscle	Origin	Insertion	Action	Innervation
Jaw-closing muscles				
Masseter (superficial and deep)	Zygomatic process of the maxilla; Zygomatic arch	External surface of the angle and ramus of the mandible; Coronoid process of the mandible	Elevates the mandible; Superficial: helps protrude the mandible; Deep: contributes to retraction of the mandible	Mandibular branch of the trigeminal nerve (cranial nerve V)
Temporalis (anterior, middle, and posterior)	Temporal fossa of the parietal and temporal bones	Coronoid process of the mandible; Anterior surface of the ramus of the mandible	Contraction of anterior and middle fibers elevates mandible; Contraction of posterior fibers may elevate and retract mandible; Unilateral contraction may contribute to lateral movement of mandible	Temporal nerve of the mandibular branch of the trigeminal nerve (cranial nerve V)
Medial (internal) pterygoid	Lateral pterygoid plate; Pterygoid fossa; Pyramidal process of the palatine bone	Internal surface of the angle and ramus of the mandible	Elevates the mandible with temporalis and masseter muscles; Protrudes mandible with lateral pterygoid muscle; Unilateral contracting: moves jaw laterally (opposite side)	Medial pterygoid nerve of the mandibular branch of the trigeminal nerve (cranial nerve V)
Jaw-opening muscles				
Lateral (external) pterygoid	Superior: greater wing of sphenoid; Inferior: lateral pterygoid plate of the sphenoid and tuberosity of the maxilla	Articular disc of the temporomandibular joint; Condyle of the mandible	Superior: co-activated with jaw-closing muscles; Inferior: bilateral contraction protrudes mandible; Unilateral contraction: moves mandible laterally toward the opposite side (grinding)	Mandibular branch of the trigeminal nerve (cranial nerve V)
Digastric	Posterior belly: mastoid process of temporal bone; Anterior belly: internal surface of mandible	Loop-shaped intermediate tendon linked to hyoid bone	Posterior belly: with the mandible stabilized, pulls the hyoid bone upward and backward, which is necessary for swallowing; Anterior belly: opens jaw when the hyoid bone is fixed	Posterior belly: digastric branch of the facial nerve (cranial nerve VII); Anterior belly: mylohyoid nerve of the mandibular branch of the trigeminal nerve (cranial nerve V) via the mylohyoid nerve
Mylohyoid	On the mylohyoid line (internal oblique line) on the internal surface of the mandible	Anterior and middle fibers: midline raphe, where fibers are linked with those of the opposite side; Posterior fibers: body of the hyoid bone	Elevates the floor of the mouth, the hyoid bone, and the tongue; Contributes to jaw opening if hyoid bone is fixed	Mylohyoid branch of the inferior alveolar nerve of the mandibular branch of the trigeminal nerve (cranial nerve V)
Geniohyoid	Internal surface of the mandibular symphysis	Anterior surface of the body of the hyoid bone	Contributes to jaw opening if hyoid bone is fixed	First cervical spinal nerve (C1) traveling with fibers of the hypoglossal nerve (cranial nerve XII)

Muscles of the Soft Palate (see Figure 3-23, p. 151)

Muscle	Origin	Insertion	Action	Innervation
Levator veli palatini	Petrous portion of temporal bone Inferior aspect of the cartilaginous eustachian tube	Palatine raphe (aponeurosis)	Elevates the soft palate	Spinal accessory nerve (cranial nerve XI) via the pharyngeal branch of the vagus nerve (cranial nerve X) and the pharyngeal plexus
Tensor veli palatini	Medial pterygoid plate Scaphoid fossa Spine of the sphenoid Lateral cartilaginous walls of the eustachian tube	By tendon around the palatine raphe (aponeurosis) and the horizontal plates of the palatine bone	Dilates the eustachian tube during swallowing and yawning May also tense the palate (on both sides)	Mandibular branch of the trigeminal nerve (cranial nerve V)
Palatoglossus (forms palatoglossal arch)	Inferior surface of the palatine raphe (aponeurosis)	Transverse and posterolateral muscular portions of the tongue	Lifts the tongue and pulls it backward Constricts the posterior limits of the oral cavity (to isolate from oropharynx)	Spinal accessory nerve (cranial nerve XI) via the pharyngeal branch of the vagus nerve (cranial nerve X) and the pharyngeal plexus
Palatopharyngeus (forms palatopharyngeal arch)	Palatine raphe (aponeurosis)	Posterior border of thyroid cartilage Inferior portion of pharynx	Pulls the soft palate down Lifts the pharynx and the larynx Directs the bolus into the pharynx during swallowing	Spinal accessory nerve (cranial nerve XI) via the pharyngeal branch of the vagus nerve (cranial nerve X) and the pharyngeal plexus
Uvular	Posterior nasal spine Palatine raphe	Uvula	May play role in elevation of the soft palate	Spinal accessory nerve (cranial nerve XI) via the pharyngeal plexus of the vagus nerve (cranial nerve X) and the pharyngeal plexus

Muscles of the Pharynx (see Figure 3-24, p. 154)

Muscle	Origin	Insertion	Action	Innervation
Superior pharyngeal constrictor	Tube starting at level of the pterygomandibular raphe	Median pharyngeal raphe	Reduces pharyngeal diameter during swallowing (propulsive pressure acting on bolus) and assists in velopharyngeal closure	Spinal accessory nerve (cranial nerve XI) via the pharyngeal branch of the vagus nerve (cranial nerve X) and the pharyngeal plexus
Middle pharyngeal constrictor	Great horns of the hyoid bone and stylohyoid ligament	Median pharyngeal raphe	Reduces pharyngeal diameter during swallowing (propulsive pressure acting on bolus)	Spinal accessory nerve (cranial nerve XI) via the pharyngeal branch of the vagus nerve (cranial nerve X) and the pharyngeal plexus
Inferior pharyngeal constrictor	Some fibers (cricopharyngeus muscle) originate from cricoid cartilage Most originate from thyroid lamina	Median pharyngeal raphe	Reduces the diameter of the inferior portions of the pharynx and acts as the sphincter-like opening (cricopharyngeus muscle) to the cervical esophagus during swallowing	Spinal accessory nerve (cranial nerve XI) via the pharyngeal branch of the vagus nerve (cranial nerve X) and the pharyngeal plexus, as well as recurrent laryngeal nerve and external branch of the superior laryngeal nerve of the vagus nerve (cranial nerve X)
Salpingopharyngeus muscle	Inferoposterior surface of the cartilage of the eustachian tube	Lateral walls of the pharynx (fibers mix with palatopharyngeus)	Contributes to elevation of the pharynx during swallowing and may contribute to the distortion of the tubal cartilage of the eustachian tube to permit aeration of the middle ear	Spinal accessory nerve (cranial nerve XI) via the pharyngeal branch of the vagus (cranial nerve X) and the pharyngeal plexus
Stylopharyngeus muscle	Base of the styloid process of the temporal bone	Mucous membrane of the pharynx and on the thyroid cartilage	Elevates the larynx and elevates and expands the pharynx during swallowing	Glossopharyngeal nerve (cranial nerve IX)

AUDITORY SYSTEM

4

■ OVERVIEW

Hearing is vital to spoken language perception and production. Hearing impairment can drastically affect speech and language development in the infant and child. In the adult, hearing is an extremely important feedback source for appropriate speech sound production. It is also extremely important for many other aspects of day-to-day living, including the perception of music and other environmental sounds. Hearing is thus a crucial function that affects many aspects of quality of life in addition to its role in speech and language.

The study of the anatomy and function of the peripheral hearing system is typically divided into three functional components: (1) the outer ear, (2) middle ear, and (3) inner ear. Each of these components serves a different but complementary role in the transduction of environmental acoustic vibrations into neural impulses (sound).

The role of the external or outer ear is to capture sounds and direct them to a membrane that converts acoustic vibrations to mechanical energy. The membrane and three attached small bones and supporting muscles and ligaments in the middle ear transmit these sounds to the sensory end organ of hearing in the inner ear. They also provide an important impedance matching function between airborne sounds in the environment and fluid vibrations in the inner ear. In the inner ear, differences in stiffness along the basilar membrane cause it to vibrate with the greatest amplitude at different places along its length for different frequencies of sound. This stimulates complex and delicate sensory receptors, which transduce the motion into neural activity in the auditory nerve and higher levels of the central auditory system.

This chapter covers these three functional components of the peripheral hearing system—the outer ear, middle ear, and inner ear—and the central auditory pathway.

■ ANATOMICAL DIVISIONS OF THE EAR (Figure 4-1)

The ear is divided into the following three major sections:
1. The outer ear is composed of the pinna and external auditory meatus.
2. The middle ear is composed of the tympanic cavity and the middle ear ossicles.
3. The inner ear is composed of the cochlea and the vestibular system.

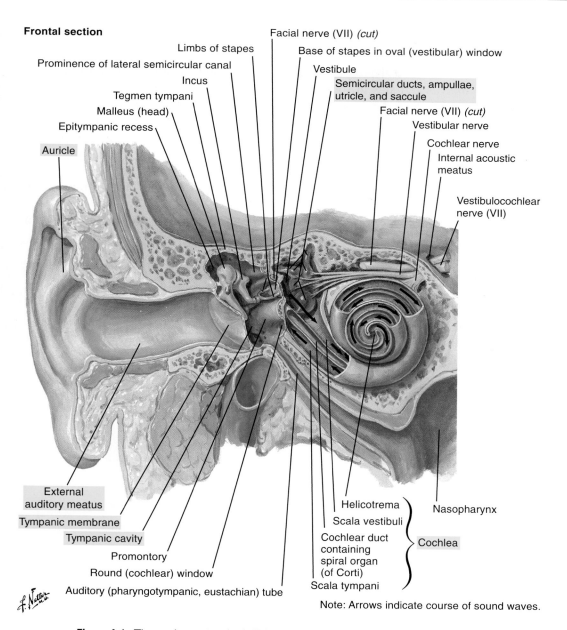

Frontal section

Facial nerve (VII) *(cut)*

Limbs of stapes

Base of stapes in oval (vestibular) window

Prominence of lateral semicircular canal

Vestibule

Incus

Semicircular ducts, ampullae, utricle, and saccule

Tegmen tympani

Malleus (head)

Facial nerve (VII) *(cut)*

Epitympanic recess

Vestibular nerve

Auricle

Cochlear nerve

Internal acoustic meatus

Vestibulocochlear nerve (VII)

External auditory meatus

Helicotrema

Nasopharynx

Tympanic membrane

Scala vestibuli

Tympanic cavity

Cochlear duct containing spiral organ (of Corti)

Cochlea

Promontory

Round (cochlear) window

Scala tympani

Auditory (pharyngotympanic, eustachian) tube

Note: Arrows indicate course of sound waves.

Figure 4-1. The main anatomical divisions of the outer, middle, and inner ear.

Legends and labels of certain figures are highlighted in yellow to emphasize the related elements in the corresponding text.

Outer Ear

Auricle or Pinna (Figure 4-2; see also Figure 4-1, p. 173)

The auricle, or pinna, is a flaplike structure that helps direct sound waves into the external auditory meatus and aids in sound localization. Some animals can move their pinna extensively for additional directional selectivity. It is composed of fibrocartilage covered by skin and attached to the temporal bone by several extrinsic muscles and ligaments. Internal ligaments and muscles join auricular structures. The following are prominent surface landmarks:

- Helix is the curved outer rim.
- Crus of the helix divides the concha, with the inferior portion being the entrance to the external auditory meatus.
- Auricular tubercle (of Darwin) is a small projection sometimes found on the lateral border of the helix.
- Antihelix is a second semicircular ridge anterior to the helix.
- Triangular fossa lies between the two crura of the antihelix.
- Scaphoid fossa lies between the helix and the antihelix.
- Tragus is the flap partially covering the entrance to the external auditory meatus.
- Antitragus is the smaller flap opposite the tragus.
- Lobule of the auricle (earlobe) is the noncartilaginous and highly vascular inferior extremity.

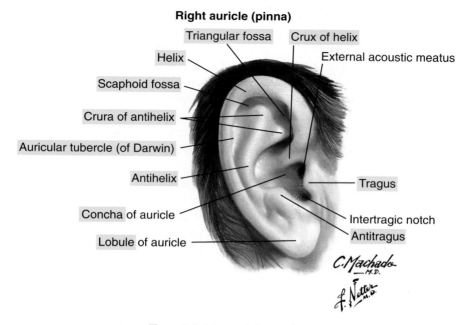

Right auricle (pinna)

Triangular fossa

Crux of helix

External acoustic meatus

Helix

Scaphoid fossa

Crura of antihelix

Auricular tubercle (of Darwin)

Antihelix

Tragus

Concha of auricle

Intertragic notch

Antitragus

Lobule of auricle

Figure 4-2. The auricle, or pinna.

External Auditory (Acoustic) Meatus or Ear Canal

The external auditory meatus, or ear canal, is an oval, S-shaped tube approximately 25 to 35 mm long and approximately 6 to 8 mm in diameter. The lateral third is cartilage and continuous with the cartilage of the auricle. The medial two-thirds are osseous. It contains cilia and glands that produce wax (ceruminous glands) and oils (sebaceous glands), and these keep the external auditory meatus clean and supple. These substances also help, in combination with the shape of the tube, to prevent foreign bodies, such as insects, from entering the canal. The resonating frequencies of the tube are such that sensitivity is increased to sounds between approximately 1000 and 6000 Hz.

Tympanic Membrane, Tympanum, or Eardrum (Figure 4-3)

The eardrum is a very thin but resilient membrane that vibrates in response to acoustic energy. It sits obliquely at the end of the external auditory meatus. It is approximately 10 mm in diameter and roughly circular in shape; its thickened outer ring (annulus) attaches to a groove in the tympanic cavity (tympanic sulcus). The normal appearance of the tympanic membrane (e.g., during visual inspection with an otoscope) is concave, smooth, and translucent. An important landmark, the "cone of light," can normally be seen radiating from a central depression called the *umbo*, which is formed by the attachment of the manubrium of the malleus (a middle ear ossicle). The process of the malleus can be seen extending toward the superior border.

The tympanic membrane has the following three layers (see Figure 4-3, *top*):

1. The outer cutaneous layer is a thin layer continuous with the lining of the external auditory meatus.
2. The middle fibrous layer is more substantial and composed of circular and radial fibers. It is deficient at the superior border, which creates the pars flaccida. The rest of the membrane is the pars tensa.
3. The internal mucous layer is continuous with the lining of the middle ear cavity.

Coronal oblique section of external acoustic meatus and middle ear (tympanic cavity)

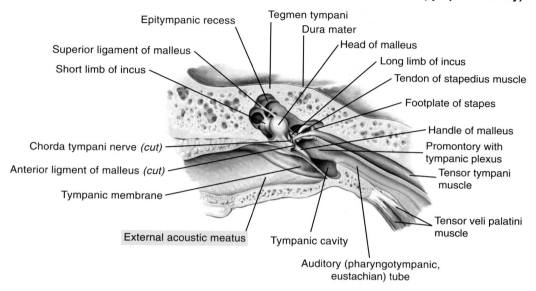

Epitympanic recess
Tegmen tympani
Dura mater
Superior ligament of malleus
Short limb of incus
Head of malleus
Long limb of incus
Tendon of stapedius muscle
Footplate of stapes
Chorda tympani nerve *(cut)*
Anterior ligament of malleus *(cut)*
Tympanic membrane
Handle of malleus
Promontory with tympanic plexus
Tensor tympani muscle
External acoustic meatus
Tympanic cavity
Auditory (pharyngotympanic, eustachian) tube
Tensor veli palatini muscle

Otoscopic view of right tympanic membrane

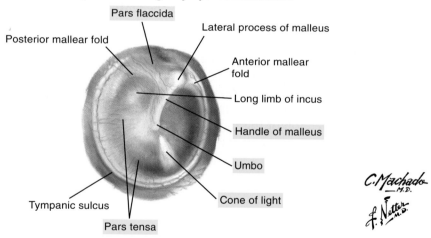

Pars flaccida
Lateral process of malleus
Posterior mallear fold
Anterior mallear fold
Long limb of incus
Handle of malleus
Umbo
Cone of light
Tympanic sulcus
Pars tensa

C. Machado — M.D.
F. Netter M.D.

Figure 4-3. The external acoustic (auditory) meatus *(top)* and tympanic membrane *(bottom)*.

Middle Ear

Tympanic Cavity (Figure 4-4; see also Figures 4-1 [p. 173] and 4-3 [p. 177, *top*])

A roughly rectangular air-filled cavity (box), the tympanic cavity lies medial to the tympanic membrane within the petrous portion of the temporal bone. It is formed by two cavities: (1) the epitympanic recess and (2) the tympanic cavity proper.

Epitympanic Recess

The epitympanic recess is superior to the tympanic membrane. It contains the head of the malleus and most of the incus.

Tympanic Cavity Proper

The tympanic cavity is the "box" containing the middle ear ossicular system and points of communication with the inner ear and auditory tube. The tegmental (superior) wall, or roof, is a thin plate of bone separating the tympanic cavity from the cranium and is called the *tegmen tympani*. The jugular (inferior) wall, or floor, is a thin bone that separates the tympanic cavity from the internal jugular vein. The tympanic nerve, a branch of the glossopharyngeal nerve (cranial nerve XI), passes through the floor of the tympanic cavity.

The membranous (lateral) wall is the tympanic membrane. The labyrinthine (medial) walls are the oval window (fenestra vestibule) and below, the round window (fenestra rotunda). Superior to the oval window passes the chorda tympani nerve (a branch of the facial [VII] cranial nerve). The carotid (anterior) wall separates the tympanic cavity from the carotid artery. Superiorly, a canal houses the tensor tympani muscle (superiorly) and more inferiorly, the opening of the eustachian tube connects the tympanic cavity to the nasopharynx (see later).

The mastoid (posterior) wall on the posterosuperior border is the mastoid antrum, a sinus with several openings to the mastoid air cells. It provides a path of direct communication between air cells and the tympanic cavity, as well as a potential path for the life-threatening infection, mastoiditis. Inferior to this is the pyramidal eminence, the point of emergence of the tendon of the stapedial muscle. Lateral to this is the chordal eminence, the point of emergence of the chorda tympani nerve into the tympanic cavity.

Lateral wall of tympanic cavity: medial (internal) view

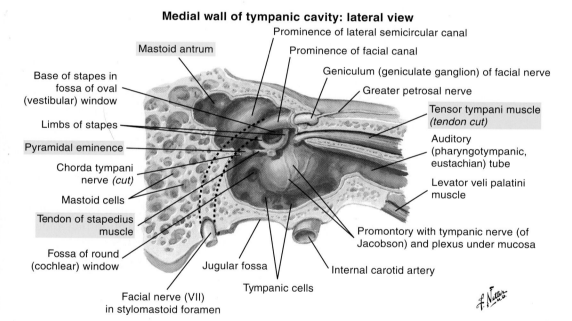

Head of malleus

Superior ligament of malleus

Epitympanic recess

Superior ligament of incus

Anterior process of malleus

Short limb of incus

Chorda tympani nerve

Posterior mallear fold

Anterior mallear fold

Posterior ligament of incus

Tensor tympani muscle

Long limb of incus

Handle of malleus

Chorda tympani nerve

Tympanic membrane
(pars tensa)

Lenticular process of incus

Auditory
(pharyngotympanic,
eustachian) tube

Facial nerve (VII)

Internal carotid artery

Medial wall of tympanic cavity: lateral view

Prominence of lateral semicircular canal

Mastoid antrum

Prominence of facial canal

Base of stapes in
fossa of oval
(vestibular) window

Geniculum (geniculate ganglion) of facial nerve

Greater petrosal nerve

Limbs of stapes

Tensor tympani muscle
(tendon cut)

Pyramidal eminence

Auditory
(pharyngotympanic,
eustachian) tube

Chorda tympani
nerve (cut)

Levator veli palatini
muscle

Mastoid cells

Tendon of stapedius
muscle

Promontory with tympanic nerve (of
Jacobson) and plexus under mucosa

Fossa of round
(cochlear) window

Jugular fossa

Internal carotid artery

Tympanic cells

Facial nerve (VII)
in stylomastoid foramen

Figure 4-4. The tympanic cavity.

Middle Ear Ossicles (Figure 4-5; see also Figure 4-4, p. 179).

The tympanic cavity proper houses the middle ear ossicles and their supporting ligaments and muscles. This system transmits acoustic vibrations from the tympanic membrane to the inner ear. Cartilaginous synovial joints connect the three ossicles.

Malleus ("Hammer"). The malleus, or "hammer," is the largest (but still only 9 mm long) and most lateral of the middle ear ossicles. It is suspended in the tympanic cavity by three ligaments; the most significant is the anterior ligament of the malleus. The manubrium (handle) is attached to the tympanic membrane. The tendon of the tensor tympani muscle (see later) attaches to the upper portion of the manubrium.

Incus ("Anvil"). The incus, or "anvil," articulates medially with the malleus and through an inferior projection (that terminates in the lenticular process) with the stapes. It is suspended from the tympanic cavity by the posterior ligament of the incus.

Stapes ("Stirrup"). The stapes, or "stirrup," is the smallest bone in the human body. Its footplate attaches to the oval window of the cochlea by the annular ligament. The tendon of the stapedial muscle is attached to the neck of the stapes.

Middle Ear Muscles (see Figure 4-5; see also Figure 4-4, p. 179)

Tensor Tympani. The tensor tympani is a muscle contained within a bony canal above and running along the eustachian tube. Its tendon enters the tympanic cavity and attaches to the manubrium of the malleus near the tympanic membrane.

The tensor tympani is innervated by a branch of the mandibular nerve of the trigeminal nerve (cranial nerve V).

Stapedial Muscle or Stapedius. The stapedius is the smallest striated muscle in the body. Its tendon emerges from the pyramidal eminence to insert on the posterior surface of the neck of the stapes.

The stapedial muscle is innervated by the stapedial branch of the facial nerve (cranial nerve VII).

Action of the Middle Ear Muscles. Muscular contraction increases the stiffness of the ossicular chain. Reflex activation may provide some sound protection benefits against intense, low-frequency sounds (below 1 to 2 kHz). Protection against rapid-onset sounds is minimal because of reflex delays (approximately 60 to 120 ms). Activation may reduce sensitivity to self-generated vocalizations transmitted to the cochlea via bone conduction.

The acoustic reflex (AR) activation of the middle ear muscles is a diagnostic tool used in the practice of audiology to assess the function of middle ear and higher-order neural processes involved in hearing.

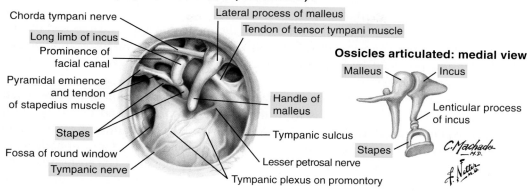

Right tympanic cavity after removal of tympanic membrane (lateral view)

Chorda tympani nerve

Long limb of incus

Prominence of facial canal

Pyramidal eminence and tendon of stapedius muscle

Stapes

Fossa of round window

Tympanic nerve

Lateral process of malleus

Tendon of tensor tympani muscle

Handle of malleus

Tympanic sulcus

Lesser petrosal nerve

Tympanic plexus on promontory

Ossicles articulated: medial view

Malleus

Incus

Lenticular process of incus

Stapes

Figure 4-5. The middle ear ossicles.

Auditory (Pharyngotympanic, Eustachian) Tube* (Figure 4-6; see Figure 4-4, p. 179).*
The pharyngotympanic, or eustachian or auditory, tube is approximately 35 to 38 mm long and extends downward, forward, and medially from the tympanic cavity to the nasopharynx. The lateral portion is osseous, and the medial portion is composed of cartilage and other connective tissue. It is normally closed by elastic recoil forces (and potentially by tension provided by muscles such as the salpingopharyngeus) to protect the middle ear from pathogens.

The tube opens during swallowing and yawning, principally by action of the tensor veli palatini with potential contributions from the levator veli palatini and tensor tympani muscles. It equalizes pressure between the middle ear and external atmospheric pressure and allows the tympanic membrane to operate efficiently in a variety of atmospheric pressures. This tube also drains the middle ear cavity and aerates tissues. The eustachian tube is shorter and more horizontally placed in children and thus provides a more direct path for middle ear infections such as otitis media.

Auditory (Pharyngotympanic, Eustachian) Tube

Cartilaginous part of auditory (pharyngotympanic, eustachian) tube at base of skull: inferior view

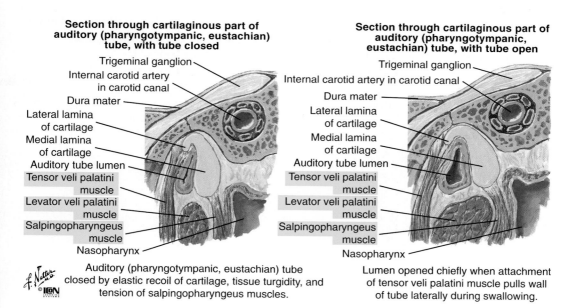

Pterygoid hamulus and medial pterygoid plate

Lateral pterygoid plate

Scaphoid fossa

Foramen ovale

Foramen spinosum

Spine of sphenoid bone

Internal carotid artery entering carotid canal

Mastoid process

Palatine process of maxilla

Horizontal plate of palatine bone

Choana

Lateral lamina } of cartilaginous part of auditory (pharyngotympanic, eustachian) tube
Medial lamina }

Foramen lacerum

Petrous part of temporal bone

Occipital condyle

Foramen magnum

Section through cartilaginous part of auditory (pharyngotympanic, eustachian) tube, with tube closed

Trigeminal ganglion
Internal carotid artery in carotid canal
Dura mater
Lateral lamina of cartilage
Medial lamina of cartilage
Auditory tube lumen
Tensor veli palatini muscle
Levator veli palatini muscle
Salpingopharyngeus muscle
Nasopharynx

Auditory (pharyngotympanic, eustachian) tube closed by elastic recoil of cartilage, tissue turgidity, and tension of salpingopharyngeus muscles.

Section through cartilaginous part of auditory (pharyngotympanic, eustachian) tube, with tube open

Trigeminal ganglion
Internal carotid artery in carotid canal
Dura mater
Lateral lamina of cartilage
Medial lamina of cartilage
Auditory tube lumen
Tensor veli palatini muscle
Levator veli palatini muscle
Salpingopharyngeus muscle
Nasopharynx

Lumen opened chiefly when attachment of tensor veli palatini muscle pulls wall of tube laterally during swallowing.

Figure 4-6. The auditory (pharyngotympanic, eustachian) tube.

Inner Ear and Vestibular System

The inner ear and vestibular system comprise the organs of hearing and equilibrium. There are two labyrinthine ("mazelike") systems: (1) the bony (osseous) outer labyrinth and (2) the internal membranous labyrinth.

Osseous or Bony Labyrinth (Figures 4-7, 4-8 [p. 186], and 4-9 [p. 187]; see Figures 4-1 [p. 173] and 4-4 [p. 179])

The bony labyrinth is composed of a series of ducts and cavities within the petrous portion of the temporal bone. It contains the vestibule, the semicircular canals, and the coiled cochlea and is composed of tissue denser than the surrounding temporal bone. Imagine pouring wax into the bony labyrinth and chipping away the "mold" to reveal the harder bony "cast" of the cochlea.

Semicircular Canals

The semicircular canals are the lateral-most portion of the bony labyrinth. Superior, posterior, and lateral canals are oriented roughly orthogonally. They are involved in balance and body orientation.

Vestibule

The vestibule is interposed between the cochlea and the semicircular canals. The oval window is the entrance to the cochlea and point of attachment of the footplate of the stapes.

Cochlea

The cochlea is the medial-most portion of the bony labyrinth. This cavity is approximately 35 mm long and coiled around a central core of bone called the *modiolus*. It is approximately two and three-quarter turns from the base (basal turn) to the apex. Small perforations in the modiolus and projecting shelf (osseous spiral lamina) allow passage of auditory nerve fibers that innervate the sensory end organs of hearing. The round window has a membranous covering that provides a point of expansion for fluid movements within the cochlea.

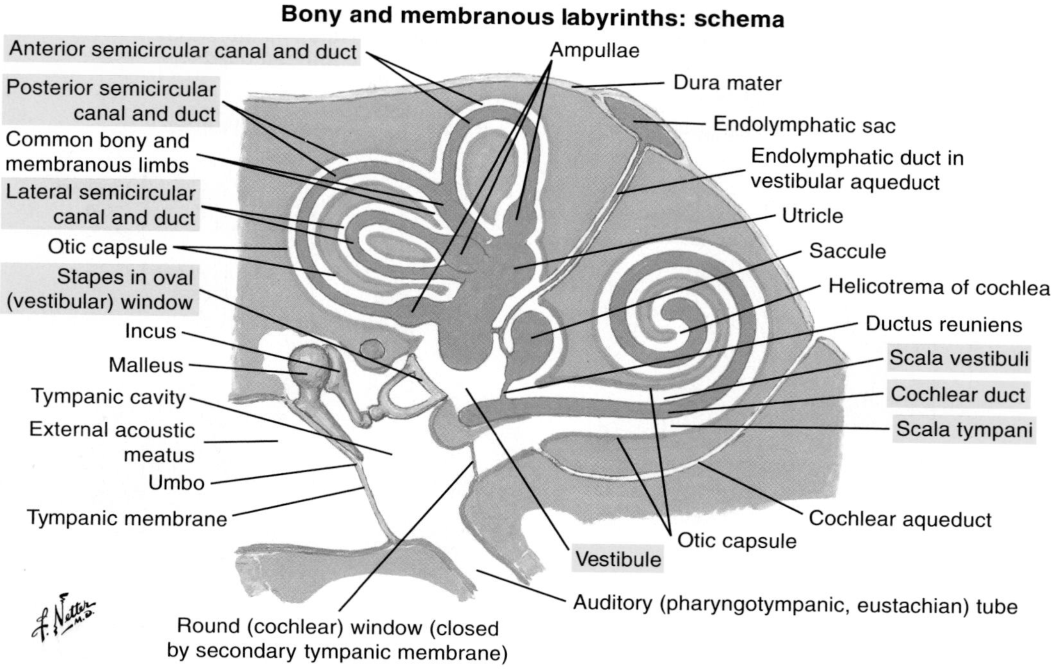

Bony and membranous labyrinths: schema

Anterior semicircular canal and duct
Posterior semicircular canal and duct
Common bony and membranous limbs
Lateral semicircular canal and duct
Otic capsule
Stapes in oval (vestibular) window
Incus
Malleus
Tympanic cavity
External acoustic meatus
Umbo
Tympanic membrane
Round (cochlear) window (closed by secondary tympanic membrane)

Ampullae
Dura mater
Endolymphatic sac
Endolymphatic duct in vestibular aqueduct
Utricle
Saccule
Helicotrema of cochlea
Ductus reuniens
Scala vestibuli
Cochlear duct
Scala tympani
Cochlear aqueduct
Otic capsule
Vestibule
Auditory (pharyngotympanic, eustachian) tube

Figure 4-7. Schema of the bony and membranous labyrinths of the inner ear.

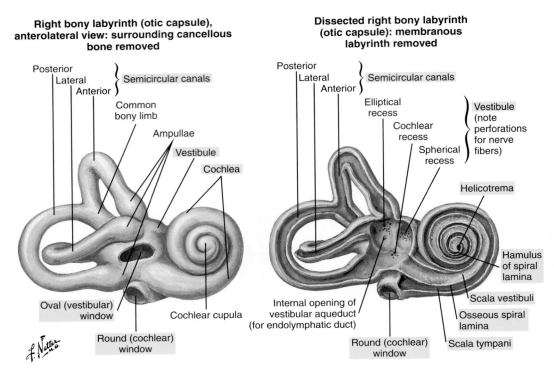

Figure 4-8. The right bony labyrinth of the inner ear.

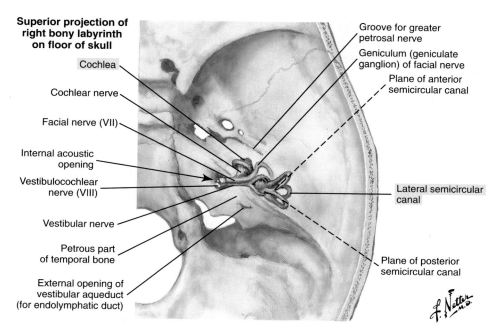

Superior projection of right bony labyrinth on floor of skull

Cochlea

Cochlear nerve

Facial nerve (VII)

Internal acoustic opening

Vestibulocochlear nerve (VIII)

Vestibular nerve

Petrous part of temporal bone

External opening of vestibular aqueduct (for endolymphatic duct)

Groove for greater petrosal nerve

Geniculum (geniculate ganglion) of facial nerve

Plane of anterior semicircular canal

Lateral semicircular canal

Plane of posterior semicircular canal

Figure 4-9. Orientation of the bony labyrinth in the skull.

Membranous Labyrinth (Figure 4-10; see Figures 4-7 [p. 185] and 4-11 [p. 192]).

The membranous labyrinth is suspended within the osseous labyrinth and composed of the membranous semicircular canals, vestibule, and cochlea. Details are provided for the membranous cochlea.

Membranous Cochlear Labyrinth (see Figure 4-7, p. 185).

The membranous cochlear labyrinth is a spirally arranged tube approximately 33 mm long and suspended in the osseous cochlea. The cochlear labyrinth includes the following three canals:

1. The scala vestibuli is the only canal in direct contact with the vestibule (thus its name).
2. The scala media, or cochlear duct, is enclosed between the scala vestibuli and scala tympani and contains the sensory end organ of hearing, the organ of Corti.
3. The scala tympani contains endolymph, and the scala vestibuli and scala tympani contain perilymph.

Right membranous labyrinth with nerves: posteromedial view

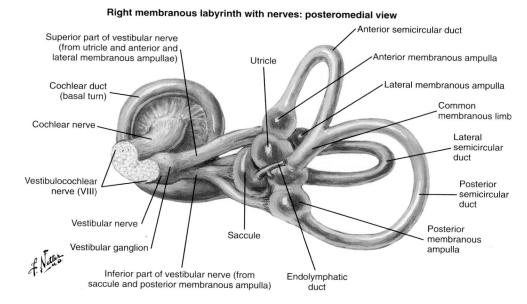

Superior part of vestibular nerve
(from utricle and anterior and
lateral membranous ampullae)

Utricle

Anterior semicircular duct

Anterior membranous ampulla

Lateral membranous ampulla

Cochlear duct
(basal turn)

Common
membranous limb

Cochlear nerve

Lateral
semicircular
duct

Vestibulocochlear
nerve (VIII)

Posterior
semicircular
duct

Vestibular nerve

Saccule

Posterior
membranous
ampulla

Vestibular ganglion

Inferior part of vestibular nerve (from
saccule and posterior membranous ampulla)

Endolymphatic
duct

Lateral projection of right membranous labyrinth

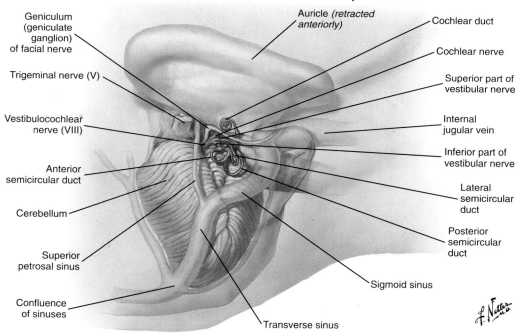

Geniculum
(geniculate
ganglion)
of facial nerve

Auricle (retracted
anteriorly)

Cochlear duct

Cochlear nerve

Trigeminal nerve (V)

Superior part of
vestibular nerve

Vestibulocochlear
nerve (VIII)

Internal
jugular vein

Inferior part of
vestibular nerve

Anterior
semicircular duct

Lateral
semicircular
duct

Cerebellum

Posterior
semicircular
duct

Superior
petrosal sinus

Confluence
of sinuses

Sigmoid sinus

Transverse sinus

Figure 4-10. The membranous labyrinth of the inner ear and its orientation in the skull.

Scala Media, or Cochlear Duct (Figures 4-11 [p. 192] and 4-12 [p. 193])

The cochlear duct is formed by the following two membranes:

1. Reissner's membrane
2. Basilar membrane

Reissner's Membrane

Reissner's membrane extends obliquely from the osseous spiral lamina to the outer bony wall and above the basilar membrane. It joins the basilar membrane at the helicotrema at the apex of the cochlea. This membrane divides the scala vestibuli from the scala media.

Basilar Membrane

The basilar membrane projects from the osseous spiral lamina and connects with the outer wall of osseous cochlea via the spiral ligament. It divides the scala media from scala tympani. Although the cross-sectional area of the bony labyrinth, or canal, becomes smaller as the apex is reached, the basilar membrane becomes wider. Thus the basilar membrane is wider and more flaccid at the apical end and narrower and stiffer at the base, and this influences its resonant properties and frequency-response characteristics. Sitting on the basilar membrane is the organ of Corti, which contains hair cells (sensory cells) and supporting cells.

Organ of Corti

The organ of Corti contains sensory (hair) cells and supporting cells.

Inner Hair Cells. One row of approximately 3500 hair cells lies along the length of the cochlea on the inner side of the tunnel of Corti. Approximately 40 stereocilia (ciliated tops of the hair cells) on each cell are arranged in parallel rows of decreasing height toward the modiolus.

Outer Hair Cells. Three to five rows of approximately 12,000 cells are present. Approximately 150 stereocilia per hair cell are arranged in the form of a V or W, with the base of the letter pointing toward the spiral ligament and with decreasing height toward the modiolus side.

Tectorial Membrane. The tectorial membrane is semitransparent and gelatinous-like. Tips of the tallest row of outer hair cell stereocilia are in contact with the tectorial membrane, which extends over hair cells from the spiral limbus.

Supporting Cells. Hair cells and their stereocilia are held in place by several supporting cells, including the inner and outer pillars or rods of Corti (forming the inner tunnel of Corti) and the inner and outer phalangeal cells. A delicate reticular lamina holds the tops of the hair cells in place and allows for shearing forces on the stereocilia by the tectorial membrane.

Section through turn of cochlea

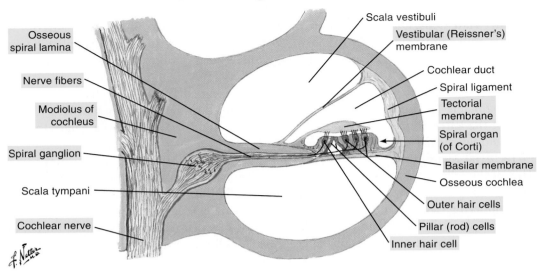

Osseous
spiral lamina

Nerve fibers

Modiolus of
cochleus

Spiral ganglion

Scala tympani

Cochlear nerve

Scala vestibuli

Vestibular (Reissner's)
membrane

Cochlear duct

Spiral ligament

Tectorial
membrane

Spiral organ
(of Corti)

Basilar membrane

Osseous cochlea

Outer hair cells

Pillar (rod) cells

Inner hair cell

Figure 4-11. Cross-section through a turn of the cochlea.

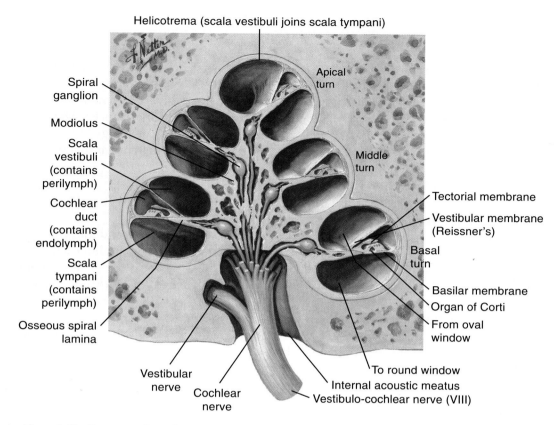

Helicotrema (scala vestibuli joins scala tympani)

Apical turn

Spiral ganglion

Modiolus

Scala vestibuli (contains perilymph)

Middle turn

Cochlear duct (contains endolymph)

Tectorial membrane

Vestibular membrane (Reissner's)

Scala tympani (contains perilymph)

Basal turn

Basilar membrane

Organ of Corti

Osseous spiral lamina

From oval window

Vestibular nerve

Cochlear nerve

To round window

Internal acoustic meatus

Vestibulo-cochlear nerve (VIII)

Figure 4-12. Cross-section of the entire cochlea. Note the scala media and cochlear nerve fibers.

■ COCHLEAR AFFERENT AND EFFERENT INNERVATION

Afferent Innervation

The cochlea is innervated by more than 30,000 sensory neurons. These eighth cranial nerve afferents convey information from the cochlea to the central nervous system. Bipolar cells have their cell bodies in spiral ganglion in the modiolus and send one process to synapse on the hair cells and a longer process (axon) to the cochlear nuclei. The process innervating the hair cells passes underneath the cells through openings in the spiral lamina called *habenula perforata*. There are two types of cochlear afferents, as follows:

1. Inner radial, or type I, fibers
2. Outer spiral, or type II, fibers

Inner Radial, or Type I, Fibers

The inner radial, or type I, fibers represent 90% to 95% of all afferents and innervate the inner hair cells exclusively. Each inner radial cell goes to one inner hair cell, but each inner hair cell receives approximately 20 inner radial fibers; this is referred to as *many to one innervation*. These fibers are called radial fibers because they fan out in a radial direction.

Outer Spiral, or Type II, Fibers

The outer spiral, or type II, fibers cross the inner tunnel of Corti and "spiral" (run longitudinally) to synapse on multiple outer hair cells. One outer spiral cell goes to many (approximately 10) outer hair cells (*one to many innervation*).

Afferent Central Auditory Pathway (Figures 4-13 [p. 196] and 4-14 [p. 197])

Afferent nerve fibers (axons) carrying sensory information from the cochlea and the semi-circular canals together form the vestibulocochlear (or auditory) nerve (cranial nerve VIII). This nerve travels through the internal auditory meatus to enter the brainstem at the medulla. Auditory nerve fibers from the cochlea first synapse onto their respective cochlear nuclei (dorsal ventral). These are referred to as *primary* or *first-order fibers*.

Beyond this lies the central auditory pathway. Fiber pathways or tracts made up of communicating axons from each ear travel ipsilaterally (on the same side) and contralaterally (on the opposite side) to higher levels of the nervous system, thus ensuring a redundancy of auditory information in the event of disease or damage.

Along the way, auditory sensory information is relayed or processed by a series of brainstem nuclei (collections of nerve cell bodies). The auditory brainstem nuclei include the superior olivary complex (in the medulla), the inferior colliculus (in the midbrain), the lateral lemniscus (in the pons), and the medial geniculate body or nucleus (thalamic auditory relay nuclei). From there, fibers are distributed (auditory radiations) to the auditory cortex located in the Sylvian fissure of the temporal lobe of each hemisphere.

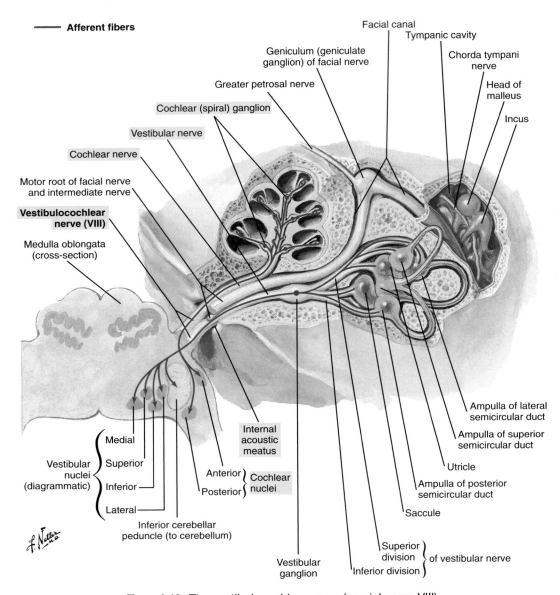

Afferent fibers

Facial canal

Tympanic cavity

Geniculum (geniculate ganglion) of facial nerve

Chorda tympani nerve

Greater petrosal nerve

Head of malleus

Cochlear (spiral) ganglion

Incus

Vestibular nerve

Cochlear nerve

Motor root of facial nerve and intermediate nerve

Vestibulocochlear nerve (VIII)

Medulla oblongata (cross-section)

Ampulla of lateral semicircular duct

Ampulla of superior semicircular duct

Internal acoustic meatus

Utricle

Medial

Vestibular nuclei (diagrammatic)

Superior

Anterior

Cochlear nuclei

Ampulla of posterior semicircular duct

Inferior

Posterior

Lateral

Saccule

Inferior cerebellar peduncle (to cerebellum)

Superior division

of vestibular nerve

Inferior division

Vestibular ganglion

Vestibular nerve

Figure 4-13. The vestibulocochlear nerve (cranial nerve VIII).

Afferent Auditory Pathways

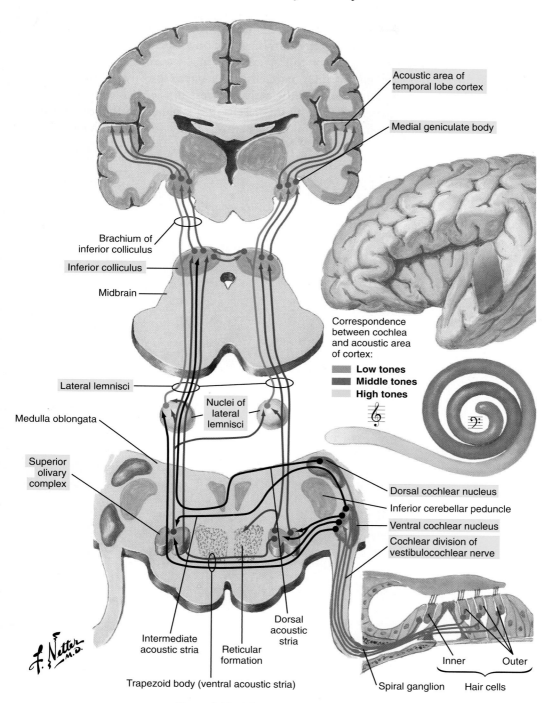

Figure 4-14. Afferent auditory pathways.

Efferent Central Auditory Pathway (Auditory Centrifugal Pathway)

A descending efferent pathway extends from the auditory cortex to the hair cells that affects the processing stages (nuclei) of the ascending system as previously described. The most well-understood part of the efferent pathway is the olivocochlear bundle, which runs from the superior olivary complex back to the hair cells in the cochlea. Medial olivocochlear bundle fibers innervate mainly outer hair cells and synapse directly on the base of the cell. This pathway may directly modulate the active process in the cochlea. Lateral olivocochlear bundle fibers innervate primarily inner cells and synapse on the afferent fibers rather than directly on the cell. The action of this pathway is not yet well understood.

NERVOUS SYSTEM

5

■ OVERVIEW

Speech production is an extremely complex sensorimotor behavior involving the coordinated action of numerous muscles distributed across several physiological systems, including the respiratory system, the laryngeal system (for phonation), and the articulation system. Multiple control mechanisms are involved in the regulation of this complex system, including a higher-order motor control system, cognitive and linguistic components interacting with brainstem and cerebellum control systems, and a feedback control system, that processes sensory information arising from various sources.

The respiratory, phonatory, and articulatory systems are also involved in deglutition. Deglutition is important for both the transportation of food and saliva and the protection of the respiratory tract during wakefulness and sleep. Like speech production, deglutition is a complex behavior that involves several levels of control, including central pattern-generating circuitry that interacts with sensory feedback and cortical control elements. Speech and deglutition appear to use a number of common control elements.

The nervous system is divided into two parts: the central nervous system (brain and spinal cord) and the peripheral nervous system (spinal and cranial nerves). This chapter first examines the structures of the central nervous system and then examines the cranial nerves because of their importance to speech, hearing, and feeding.

The brain develops from three primary structures: the rhombencephalon (or hindbrain), the mesencephalon (or midbrain), and the prosencephalon (or forebrain). The rhombencephalon in turn divides into the metencephalon (pons and cerebellum) and the myelencephalon (medulla). The prosencephalon divides into the telencephalon (cerebral hemispheres and basal ganglia) and the diencephalon (thalamus, hypothalamus, epithalamus, and subthalamus). The pons, medulla, and midbrain collectively form the *brainstem*.

**Developmental and Anatomical Divisions of the
Central Nervous System (CNS)**

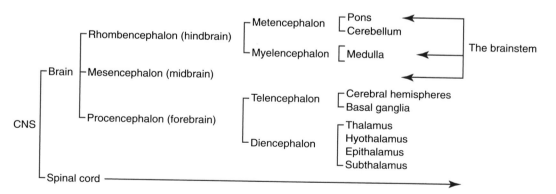

■ NEUROANATOMICAL TERMS OF DIRECTION (Figure 5-1)

When describing the location of structures in the brain, it is important to recognize that the neuroaxis flexes at the level of the midbrain during development. Thus, when speaking of the upper portions of the brainstem (above the diencephalon) and the cerebral hemi-spheres, *rostral* (or anterior) refers to the front of the brain and *caudal* (or posterior) refers to the back. *Dorsal* (or superior) is toward the top of the brain and *ventral* (or inferior) is away from the top. Because of the superior-inferior orientation of the spinal cord and the lower portions of the brainstem, the terms of direction described in the Introduction to this book apply (see Figure 5-1).

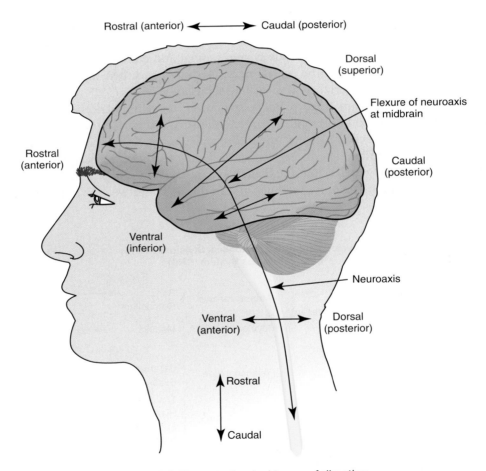

Figure 5-1 Neuroanatomical terms of direction.

■ TELENCEPHALON (CEREBRAL HEMISPHERES OR CEREBRUM AND BASAL GANGLIA)

Surface Structures

Characteristic Features

The telencephalon is composed of the two cerebral hemispheres separated by the longitudinal fissure (see Figure 5-4, p. 208). Each hemisphere is composed of numerous irregular gyri (convolutions) separated by sulci (or fissures). The cerebral hemispheres are made up of gray matter (cell bodies) and white matter (nerve fiber axons). White matter fiber tractways are categorized as to whether they project to other brain areas (projection fibers), connect different areas within a cerebral hemisphere (association fibers), or connect the two cerebral hemispheres (commissural fibers).

The cerebral cortex is the external, thin layer of gray matter capping the white matter core of the cerebral hemispheres. The cortex is stratified into six cellular layers (numbered from I to VI, starting from the most superficial layer). The laminar organization of the cortex into layers varies from region to region and reflects functional differences.

The organization of the cortical motor areas (i.e., the primary motor area, the supplementary motor area, and the lateral premotor cortex) is characterized by poor layering, such as the absence of layer IV, which contains granular cells, and the presence in layer V of giant pyramidal cells called *Betz cells*. The organization of the motor areas is referred to as *agranular*. The nonprimary motor areas (the supplementary motor area and the lateral premotor cortex) contain fewer Betz cells than the primary motor areas. The pyramidal cells contribute to two important motor pathways: (1) the corticobulbar projecting to the brainstem and cranial motoneurons and (2) the corticospinal tracts projecting to the spinal cord and spinal motoneurons. The neurons whose axons form these descending pathways are sometimes called *upper motoneurons,* whereas the cranial or spinal motoneurons they innervate are called *lower motoneurons.* Although there are other motor pathways, but the corticobulbar and corticospinal tracts have privileged access to the motoneurons of the brainstem and spinal cord, respectively.

The primary sensory areas, located just caudal to the primary motor area, have an internal organization that is referred to as *granular.* Layering of these areas is also poor but different from the layering of the agranular (motor) areas. Granular areas contain few pyramidal cells and a large number of another type of neuron called *stellar cells.* Primary sensory areas process sensory feedback, including information related to speech and other movements.

Important Sulci

The telencephalon contains the following significant sulci:

- The longitudinal fissure is also referred to as the *sagittal fissure* or *longitudinal cerebral fissure.*
- The lateral sulcus is located on the lateral surface and is also known as the *Sylvian fissure* (see Figure 5-3, p. 207).
- The central sulcus is located on the lateral surface and is also known as the *rolandic fissure* or *fissure of Rolando* (see Figure 5-3, p. 207).
- The parietooccipital sulcus is located on the medial surface (see Figure 5-2, p. 206).
- The calcarine sulcus is located on the posteriomedial surface (see Figure 5-4, p. 208).

Cerebral Lobes

The sulci are important landmarks to locate the cerebral lobes. Each hemisphere contains the following four lobes (see Figure 5-3, p. 207):

1. The frontal lobe is located rostral to the central sulcus and dorsal to the lateral sulcus.
2. The parietal lobe is caudal to the central sulcus. Its caudal limit is an imaginary extension on the lateral surface of the parietooccipital sulcus. The inferior limit is a posterior extension of the sylvian sulcus.
3. The occipital lobe is caudal to the posterior boundary of the parietal lobe, which is an extension of the parietooccipital sulcus.
4. The temporal lobe is inferior to the frontal and parietal lobes and rostral to the occipital lobe.

Internal Surface (Figure 5-2, p. 206; see also Figure 5-6, p. 211)

The third ventricle is part of the ventricular system, which is a series of ducts that are involved in the production and circulation of cerebrospinal fluid. The corpus callosum is composed of a collection of axons connecting the two hemispheres. The cingulate gyrus (or cingulum) is located above the corpus callosum. The cingulate gyrus contains a number of anatomically and functionally distinct areas. The cingulate gyrus divides at the level of the anterior commissure into a caudal and a rostral (agranular) region; the latter is involved in movement preparation. Both regions (rostral and caudal) further divide into several functionally distinct areas.

The medial segment of the superior frontal gyrus contains two important motor (agranular) areas: (1) the supplementary motor area proper and (2) the presupplementary motor area. The boundary between these areas is an imaginary line passing through the anterior commissure. Similar to the primary motor area, these areas are somatotopically organized and are involved in the production of speech and other movements, especially for selection, preparation, and initiation, and the temporal sequencing of movement components.

External Surface (Figures 5-3 [p. 207] and 5-4 [p. 208])

The following structures can be identified on the frontal lobe:

- The caudal portion of the precentral gyrus is adjacent to the central sulcus and runs from the lateral sulcus to the mediosuperior surface of the frontal lobe. It contains the agranular primary motor cortex or area. The primary motor cortex is somatotopically organized with body parts often represented by a distorted body topographical map called a *homunculus*. The face, larynx, and pharynx have a large representation on the inferior portion of the gyrus (Figure 5-5, p. 209) reflecting the precision requirements of movements of these structures for speech and feeding/swallowing (and other orofacial movements).
- The anterior portion of the precentral gyrus, near the precentral sulcus, contains the premotor cortex (lateral premotor cortex). The premotor cortex divides into a ventral and a dorsal segment, approximately at the level of the inferior frontal sulcus. Both the ventral and the dorsal premotor area further divide into functionally distinct regions. The premotor cortex is involved in the production of speech and other motor behaviors, particularly for the sensori-motor planning of movements, as well as more cognitive aspects of movement preparation such as response selection.
- The inferior frontal gyrus divides into a ventral orbital area (pars orbitalis), a caudal opercular area (pars opercularis), and a triangular area (pars triangularis). The opercular and triangular regions in the left hemisphere are collectively referred to as *Broca's area* and are important for the planning and articulation of speech (opercular), as well as for language comprehension, including semantics and syntax (triangular).

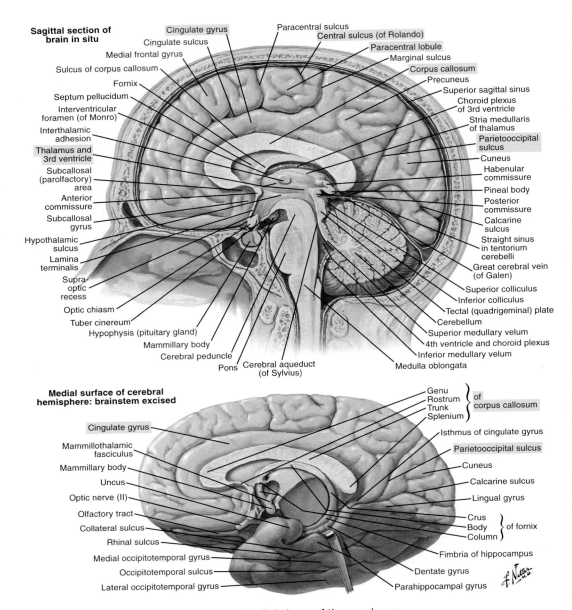

Figure 5-2 Medial views of the cerebrum.

Legends and labels of certain figures are highlighted in yellow to emphasize the related elements in the corresponding text.

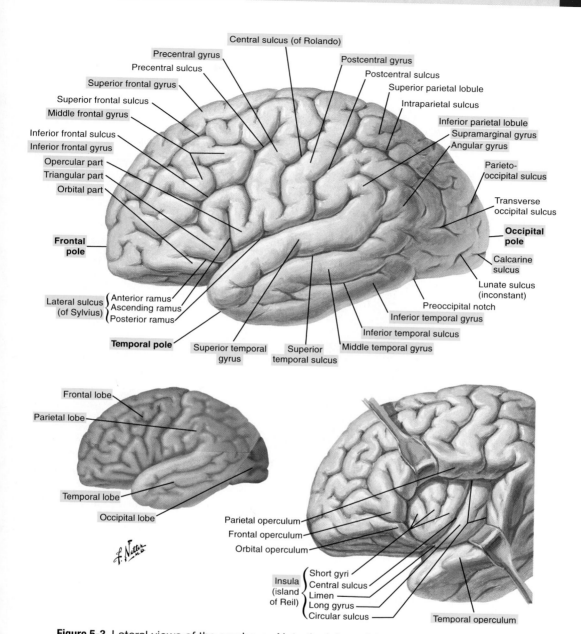

Figure 5-3 Lateral views of the cerebrum. Note the lobes of the cerebral hemispheres.

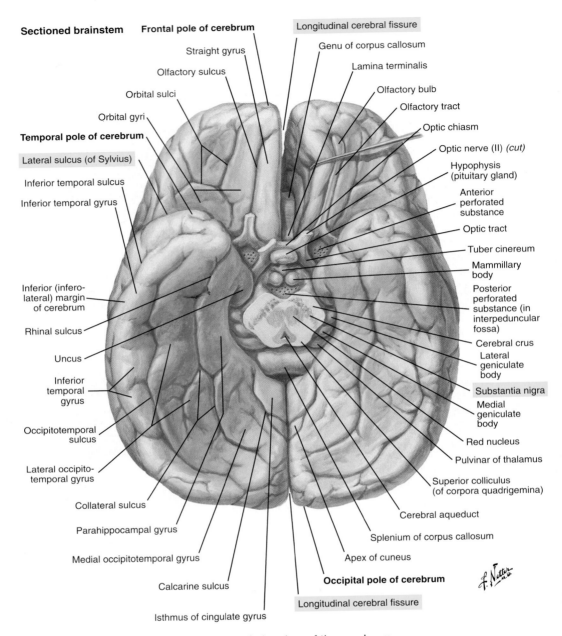

Sectioned brainstem   Frontal pole of cerebrum   Longitudinal cerebral fissure

Straight gyrus

Genu of corpus callosum

Olfactory sulcus

Lamina terminalis

Orbital sulci

Olfactory bulb

Orbital gyri

Olfactory tract

Temporal pole of cerebrum

Optic chiasm

Lateral sulcus (of Sylvius)

Optic nerve (II) (cut)

Hypophysis
(pituitary gland)

Inferior temporal sulcus

Anterior
perforated
substance

Inferior temporal gyrus

Optic tract

Tuber cinereum

Mammillary
body

Inferior (infero-
lateral) margin
of cerebrum

Posterior
perforated
substance (in
interpeduncular
fossa)

Rhinal sulcus

Cerebral crus

Uncus

Lateral
geniculate
body

Inferior
temporal
gyrus

Substantia nigra

Medial
geniculate
body

Occipitotemporal
sulcus

Red nucleus

Pulvinar of thalamus

Lateral occipito-
temporal gyrus

Superior colliculus
(of corpora quadrigemina)

Collateral sulcus

Cerebral aqueduct

Parahippocampal gyrus

Splenium of corpus callosum

Medial occipitotemporal gyrus

Apex of cuneus

Calcarine sulcus

Occipital pole of cerebrum

Longitudinal cerebral fissure

Isthmus of cingulate gyrus

Figure 5-4 Inferior view of the cerebrum.

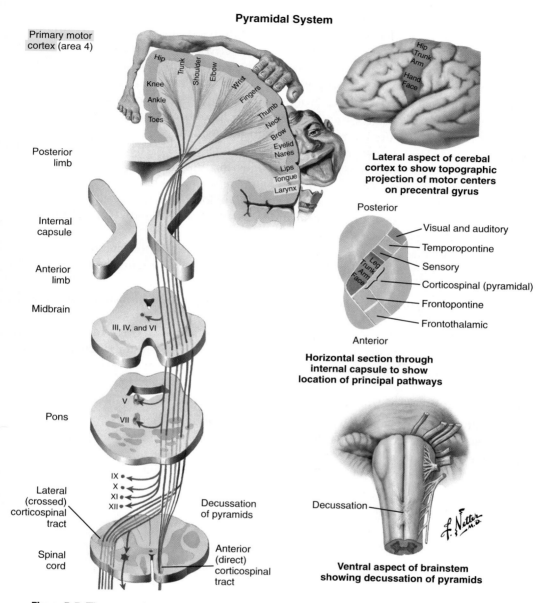

Pyramidal System

Primary motor cortex (area 4)

Hip
Trunk
Shoulder
Elbow
Knee
Wrist
Ankle
Fingers
Toes
Thumb
Neck
Brow
Eyelid
Nares
Lips
Tongue
Larynx

Posterior limb

Internal capsule

Anterior limb

Midbrain

III, IV, and VI

Pons

V

VII

IX
X
XI
XII

Lateral (crossed) corticospinal tract

Spinal cord

Decussation of pyramids

Anterior (direct) corticospinal tract

Hip
Trunk
Arm
Hand
Face

Lateral aspect of cerebral cortex to show topographic projection of motor centers on precentral gyrus

Posterior

Visual and auditory

Temporopontine

Leg
Trunk
Arm
Face

Sensory

Corticospinal (pyramidal)

Frontopontine

Frontothalamic

Anterior

Horizontal section through internal capsule to show location of principal pathways

Decussation

Ventral aspect of brainstem showing decussation of pyramids

Figure 5-5 The pyramidal system, representing the parts of the body on the motor cortex.

The following structures can be identified on the parietal lobe:
- The postcentral gyrus (located posterior or caudal to the central sulcus) is important for the processing of sensory information, thus it is called the *primary sensory (somatosensory) cortex* or *area*. Similar to the primary motor cortex, body parts are topographically represented in the primary sensory cortex.
- The supramarginal gyrus is located around the caudal border of the lateral fissure.
- The angular gyrus is located around the caudal border of the superior temporal sulcus.

These two areas, the supramarginal gyrus and the angular gyrus, receive auditory, visual, and somatosensory information. The supramarginal gyrus participates in phonological processing, and the angular gyrus is involved in semantic processing.

The following structures can be identified on the temporal lobe:
- The superior, middle, and inferior temporal gyri are located here. The *temporal operculum* is formed by the superior temporal and transverse temporal gyri. Operculum means "lid," and in this case it covers the insula.
- Heschl's gyrus (not shown in Figure 5-3) is located deep within the lateral sulcus on the temporal operculum (see Figure 5-3, p. 207). Heschl's gyrus contains the primary auditory cortex or area.
- The planum temporale is located on the temporal operculum, posterior to Heschl's gyrus.
- Wernicke's area is on the posterior half of the superior temporal gyrus of the left hemisphere and includes the planum temporale. This area is important for language, particularly for language comprehension.

Internal Structures of the Cerebral Hemispheres

Underneath the cortex, the following structures can be found:
- White matter tracts connecting different parts of the cortex or traveling to or from the brainstem and spinal cord
- The hippocampal formation, the amygdala, and the basal ganglia

Basal Ganglia (Figure 5-6)

The basal ganglia contain the following:

Anatomic structures
- Caudate nucleus
- Putamen
- Globus pallidus (external and internal segments)

Functional components
- Substantia nigra
- Subthalamic nucleus

The basal ganglia, which are located deep in the telencephalon, are also known as the *basal nuclei*. They participate in the control of body posture and muscle tonus and in planning and initiating movements. The putamen and globus pallidus are collectively referred to as the *lentiform* or *lenticular nucleus*. The caudate nucleus and the lentiform nucleus together form the *striate body* or the corpus striatum. The substantia nigra (midbrain) and subthalamic nuclei (diencephalon), although not anatomically located in the telencephalon, are often considered to be functional components of the basal ganglia.

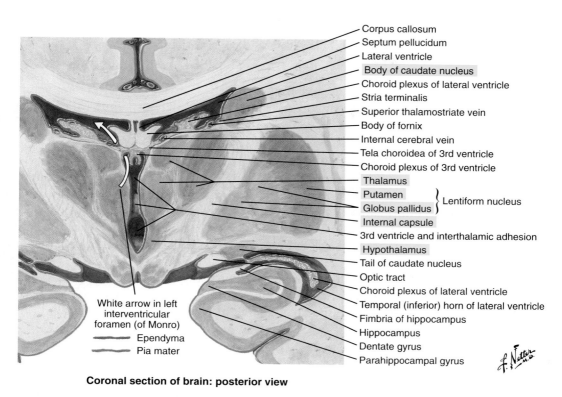

Corpus callosum
Septum pellucidum
Lateral ventricle
Body of caudate nucleus
Choroid plexus of lateral ventricle
Stria terminalis
Superior thalamostriate vein
Body of fornix
Internal cerebral vein
Tela choroidea of 3rd ventricle
Choroid plexus of 3rd ventricle
Thalamus
Putamen ⎫
Globus pallidus ⎬ Lentiform nucleus
Internal capsule ⎭
3rd ventricle and interthalamic adhesion
Hypothalamus
Tail of caudate nucleus
Optic tract
Choroid plexus of lateral ventricle
Temporal (inferior) horn of lateral ventricle
Fimbria of hippocampus
Hippocampus
Dentate gyrus
Parahippocampal gyrus

White arrow in left
interventricular
foramen (of Monro)
━━━ Ependyma
━━━ Pia mater

Coronal section of brain: posterior view

Figure 5-6 A coronal section of the basal ganglia, thalamus, and associated structures.

■ DIENCEPHALON (THALAMUS, HYPOTHALAMUS, EPITHALAMUS, AND SUBTHALAMUS) (see Figure 5-6, p. 211)

Characteristic Features

The diencephalon is located deep to and almost entirely encircled by the cerebral hemispheres. It contains the following structures: (1) thalamus, (2) hypothalamus, (3) epithalamus, and (4) subthalamus.

Importance for Speech and Swallowing

The thalamus contains multiple nuclei that are part of motor, sensory, and associative pathways. The thalamus receives all sensory feedback, with the exception of olfactory feedback, and relays this information to the cortex. Because of this, it is often considered only as sensory relay nuclei. However, the thalamus has reciprocal connections with the cortex, receiving not only sensory feedback but motor signals, indicating an additional role in movement production.

The ventrolateral nucleus and the ventroanterior nucleus connect the basal ganglia and cerebellum to their respective motor and premotor cortices and are consequently involved in motor planning and initiation of speech and other movements.

■ MESENCEPHALON (MIDBRAIN) (see Figures 5-2 [p. 206] and 5-4 [p. 208])

Characteristic Features

The mesencephalon is the smallest portion of the brainstem and is located just above the pons. It contains a number of nuclei, including the substantia nigra (part of the basal ganglia) and the inferior and superior colliculi, which are collectively referred to as the *corpora quadrigemina*. Inferior colliculi are important central auditory pathway nuclei, and the superior colliculi are important central visual pathway nuclei.

Fibers from the corticospinal, corticobulbar, and corticopontine tracts pass through the mesencephalon. The base of the mesencephalon includes the superior cerebellar peduncles.

Importance for Speech and Swallowing

The substantia nigra has an important role in regulating motor activity, particularly in initiating and terminating movements. The mesencephalon houses the nuclei of several cranial nerves (see section on Cranial Nerves). The inferior colliculi are important auditory relay and processing nuclei.

■ METENCEPHALON (PONS AND CEREBELLUM) (Figure 5-7; see also Figure 5-2, p. 206)

Characteristic Features

The metencephalon is composed of the pons and cerebellum (discussed in more detail later). The pons contains vertical and horizontal fibers. The horizontal fibers are located on the anterior surface of the pons and form the cerebellar peduncles, which connect the brainstem to the cerebellum. The vertical (longitudinal) fibers of the metencephalon are continuous with the myelencephalon longitudinal fibers and carry sensory and motor information.

Importance for Speech and Swallowing

The pons contains the motor nuclei of two cranial nerves important for speech and swallowing: the trigeminal nerve (V) and the facial nerve (VII).

■ MYELENCEPHALON (MEDULLA OBLONGATA) (Figure 5-7; see also Figure 5-2, p. 206)

Characteristic Features

The medulla is the most caudal portion of the brainstem. It is located between the pons and the spinal cord, ventral to the cerebellum. The medulla resembles an enlargement of the spinal cord.

Importance for Speech and Swallowing

The medulla contains the nucleus ambiguus, which contains the motor nuclei of cranial nerves important for speech and swallowing: the glossopharyngeal (IV), the vagus (X), and the accessory (XI) nerves. The nucleus ambiguus receives inputs primarily from the contralateral hemisphere.

Brainstem Pattern-Generating Circuitry

The pons and medulla contain important pattern-generating nuclei, sometimes called brainstem *central pattern generators (CPGs)*. This term is used because these collections of neurons contain the neural circuitry needed to generate some fundamental rhythmic and repetitive movements such as locomotion, mastication, swallowing, and respiration. The pattern generators for these movements may share multifunctional neurons that are biased to produce one or the other behavior (or coordinate the two, in the case of breathing and swallowing, for example). Although basic patterns can be generated by brainstem nuclei alone, adapting movements to changing external or internal environmental conditions requires sensory feedback and inputs from higher levels of the nervous system (e.g., cortical inputs). It has also been suggested that speech production uses or "fractionates" some of the brainstem circuitry for breathing, mastication, and swallowing for the production of speech.

Posterior phantom view

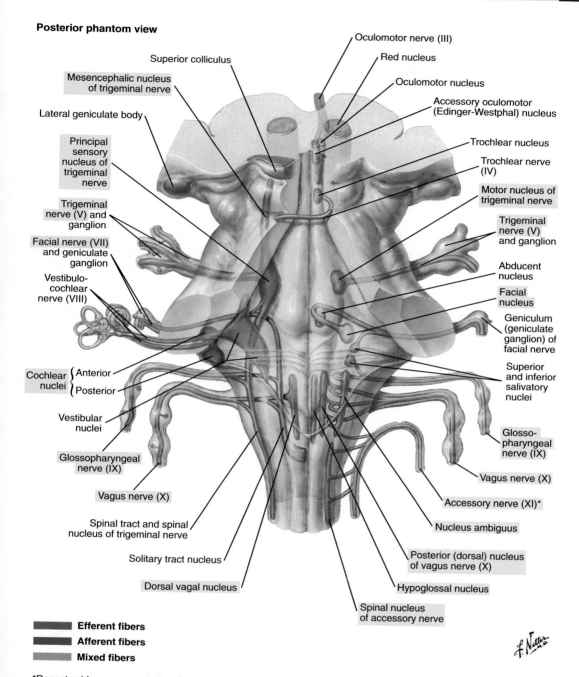

Superior colliculus

Mesencephalic nucleus
of trigeminal nerve

Lateral geniculate body

Principal
sensory
nucleus of
trigeminal
nerve

Trigeminal
nerve (V) and
ganglion

Facial nerve (VII)
and geniculate
ganglion

Vestibulo-
cochlear
nerve (VIII)

Cochlear { Anterior
nuclei { Posterior

Vestibular
nuclei

Glossopharyngeal
nerve (IX)

Vagus nerve (X)

Spinal tract and spinal
nucleus of trigeminal nerve

Solitary tract nucleus

Dorsal vagal nucleus

Oculomotor nerve (III)

Red nucleus

Oculomotor nucleus

Accessory oculomotor
(Edinger-Westphal) nucleus

Trochlear nucleus

Trochlear nerve
(IV)

Motor nucleus of
trigeminal nerve

Trigeminal
nerve (V)
and ganglion

Abducent
nucleus

Facial
nucleus

Geniculum
(geniculate
ganglion) of
facial nerve

Superior
and inferior
salivatory
nuclei

Glosso-
pharyngeal
nerve (IX)

Vagus nerve (X)

Accessory nerve (XI)*

Nucleus ambiguus

Posterior (dorsal) nucleus
of vagus nerve (X)

Hypoglossal nucleus

Spinal nucleus
of accessory nerve

■ **Efferent fibers**
■ **Afferent fibers**
■ **Mixed fibers**

*Recent evidence suggests that the accessory nerve lacks a cranial root and has no connection to the vagus nerve.
Verification of this finding awaits further investigation.

Figure 5-7 The location of the cranial nerve nuclei and fiber tracts in the brainstem.

■ SPINAL CORD (Figure 5-8)

Characteristic Features

The spinal cord is the elongated, nearly cylindrical part of the central nervous system contained within the vertebral column. The superior boundary of the spinal cord is the base of the medulla, and its inferior boundary is the first or second lumbar vertebra. The spinal cord is protected by the vertebral column and the spinal meninges. It is divided into 31 segments, and each segment gives rise to a ventral root and a dorsal root, which fuse to form a spinal nerve.

Internal Structures

In a cross-section of the spinal cord, the following structures can be seen:
- The butterfly-shaped gray matter is located deep into the cord.
- The white matter surrounds the gray matter and contains ascending and descending pathways. The white matter pathways carry information from the brain to the periphery (motor) and from the periphery to the brain (sensory).

Spinal Cord Cross-Sections: Fiber Tracts

Sections through spinal cord at various levels

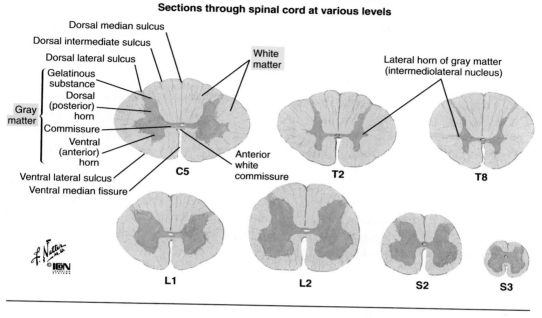

Dorsal median sulcus
Dorsal intermediate sulcus
Dorsal lateral sulcus
Gelatinous substance
Dorsal (posterior) horn
Gray matter
Commissure
Ventral (anterior) horn
Ventral lateral sulcus
Ventral median fissure

White matter

Lateral horn of gray matter (intermediolateral nucleus)

Anterior white commissure

C5   T2   T8

L1   L2   S2   S3

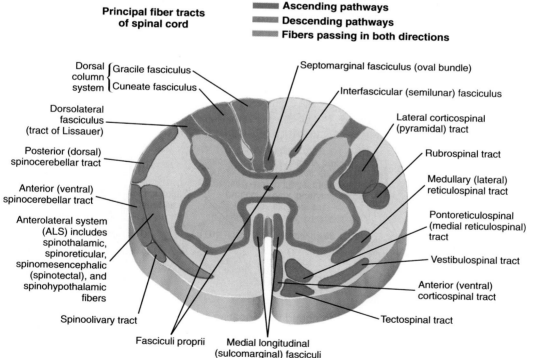

Principal fiber tracts of spinal cord

Ascending pathways
Descending pathways
Fibers passing in both directions

Dorsal column system { Gracile fasciculus, Cuneate fasciculus }
Dorsolateral fasciculus (tract of Lissauer)
Posterior (dorsal) spinocerebellar tract
Anterior (ventral) spinocerebellar tract
Anterolateral system (ALS) includes spinothalamic, spinoreticular, spinomesencephalic (spinotectal), and spinohypothalamic fibers
Spinoolivary tract

Septomarginal fasciculus (oval bundle)
Interfascicular (semilunar) fasciculus
Lateral corticospinal (pyramidal) tract
Rubrospinal tract
Medullary (lateral) reticulospinal tract
Pontoreticulospinal (medial reticulospinal) tract
Vestibulospinal tract
Anterior (ventral) corticospinal tract
Tectospinal tract

Fasciculi proprii   Medial longitudinal (sulcomarginal) fasciculi

Figure 5-8 Fiber tracts of the spinal cord.

■ CEREBELLUM (Figures 5-9 [p. 220] and 5-10 [p. 221])

Characteristic Features

The cerebellum is located posterior to the pons and medulla and inferior to the occipital lobe, which partially overlaps it. It is connected to the brainstem through three pairs of cerebellar peduncles: the inferior, middle, and superior peduncles. The external layer of the cerebellum forms the cerebellar cortex, which is made up of gray matter; the internal core of the cerebellum is made up of white matter and several deep nuclei.

The cerebellum has a midline structure called the *vermis* that connects the two cerebellar hemispheres. Each hemisphere is divided into three lobes: anterior, posterior, and flocculonodular. The cerebellum can be divided into three parts based on functional and phylogenetic (from the evolutionary oldest to the most recent) criteria: the vestibulocerebellum (or archicerebellum), the spinocerebellum (or paleocerebellum), and the cerebrocerebellum (or neocerebellum). The archicerebellum corresponds to the flocculonodular lobe; the paleocerebellum corresponds to the anterior lobe and a fraction of the posterior lobe; and the neocerebellum corresponds to the posterior lobe.

The cerebellum contains four pairs of deep nuclei embedded in white matter, which act as relay for the efferent cerebellar pathways. From lateral to medial, these nuclei are the dentate nucleus, which serves as a relay for the neocerebellum; the emboliform nucleus, which serves as a relay for the paleocerebellum; the globose nucleus, which also serves as a relay for the paleocerebellum; and the fastigial nucleus, which serves as a relay for the archicerebellum.

Importance for Speech and Swallowing

The anterior lobe and the vermis are involved in regulating posture. The posterior lobe is involved in the precise coordination of movements, such as grasping and reaching and speech. Each cerebellar region is connected to a specific part of the central nervous system.

The archicerebellum is connected to the vestibular system of the internal ear and is concerned with balance and equilibrium. The paleocerebellum, or spinocerebellum, which is mainly composed of the vermis, is connected to the spinal cord. The neocerebellum, or cerebrocerebellum, is connected to the cerebral hemispheres and is concerned with the coordination of rapid movements such as the coordination of articulation movements for speech, motor learning, and movement automaticity.

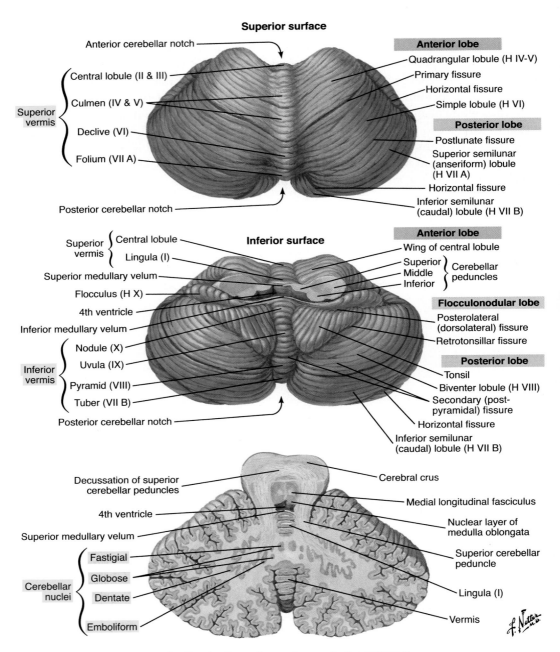

Superior surface

Anterior cerebellar notch

Anterior lobe
Quadrangular lobule (H IV-V)
Primary fissure
Horizontal fissure
Simple lobule (H VI)

Superior vermis
Central lobule (II & III)
Culmen (IV & V)
Declive (VI)
Folium (VII A)

Posterior lobe
Postlunate fissure
Superior semilunar (anseriform) lobule (H VII A)
Horizontal fissure
Inferior semilunar (caudal) lobule (H VII B)

Posterior cerebellar notch

Inferior surface

Superior vermis
Central lobule
Lingula (I)
Superior medullary velum
Flocculus (H X)
4th ventricle
Inferior medullary velum

Inferior vermis
Nodule (X)
Uvula (IX)
Pyramid (VIII)
Tuber (VII B)

Posterior cerebellar notch

Anterior lobe
Wing of central lobule
Superior
Middle
Inferior
Cerebellar peduncles

Flocculonodular lobe
Posterolateral (dorsolateral) fissure
Retrotonsillar fissure

Posterior lobe
Tonsil
Biventer lobule (H VIII)
Secondary (post-pyramidal) fissure
Horizontal fissure
Inferior semilunar (caudal) lobule (H VII B)

Decussation of superior cerebellar peduncles
4th ventricle
Superior medullary velum

Cerebellar nuclei
Fastigial
Globose
Dentate
Emboliform

Cerebral crus
Medial longitudinal fasciculus
Nuclear layer of medulla oblongata
Superior cerebellar peduncle
Lingula (I)
Vermis

Section in plane of superior cerebellar peduncle

Figure 5-9 The cerebellum.

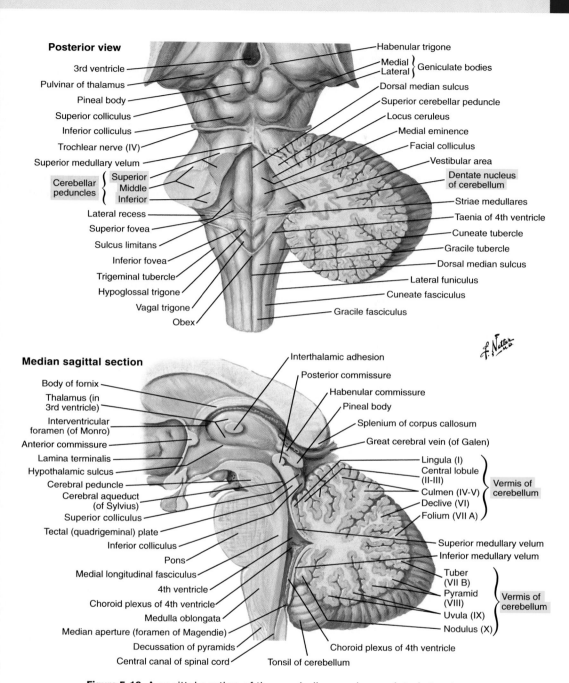

Posterior view

- Habenular trigone
- 3rd ventricle
- Pulvinar of thalamus
- Pineal body
- Superior colliculus
- Inferior colliculus
- Trochlear nerve (IV)
- Superior medullary velum
- Cerebellar peduncles { Superior Middle Inferior
- Lateral recess
- Superior fovea
- Sulcus limitans
- Inferior fovea
- Trigeminal tubercle
- Hypoglossal trigone
- Vagal trigone
- Obex

- Medial } Lateral } Geniculate bodies
- Dorsal median sulcus
- Superior cerebellar peduncle
- Locus ceruleus
- Medial eminence
- Facial colliculus
- Vestibular area
- Dentate nucleus of cerebellum
- Striae medullares
- Taenia of 4th ventricle
- Cuneate tubercle
- Gracile tubercle
- Dorsal median sulcus
- Lateral funiculus
- Cuneate fasciculus
- Gracile fasciculus

Median sagittal section

- Body of fornix
- Thalamus (in 3rd ventricle)
- Interventricular foramen (of Monro)
- Anterior commissure
- Lamina terminalis
- Hypothalamic sulcus
- Cerebral peduncle
- Cerebral aqueduct (of Sylvius)
- Superior colliculus
- Tectal (quadrigeminal) plate
- Inferior colliculus
- Pons
- Medial longitudinal fasciculus
- 4th ventricle
- Choroid plexus of 4th ventricle
- Medulla oblongata
- Median aperture (foramen of Magendie)
- Decussation of pyramids
- Central canal of spinal cord

- Interthalamic adhesion
- Posterior commissure
- Habenular commissure
- Pineal body
- Splenium of corpus callosum
- Great cerebral vein (of Galen)
- Lingula (I)
- Central lobule (II-III)
- Culmen (IV-V) } Vermis of cerebellum
- Declive (VI)
- Folium (VII A)
- Superior medullary velum
- Inferior medullary velum
- Tuber (VII B)
- Pyramid (VIII) } Vermis of cerebellum
- Uvula (IX)
- Nodulus (X)
- Choroid plexus of 4th ventricle
- Tonsil of cerebellum

Figure 5-10 A sagittal section of the cerebellum and associated structures.

■ MENINGES (Figure 5-11)

The following three layers of protective coatings surround the brain (and spinal cord):
1. Dura mater
2. Arachnoid mater
3. Pia mater

Dura Mater

The dura mater has a tough outer fibrous layer, which is actually two layers (inner meningeal and outer periosteal) that are contiguous except where they separate to accommodate the dural venous sinuses.

Arachnoid Mater

Arachnoid mater is the medial layer and is much thinner than the dura mater. It follows the convolutions of the brain but not as closely as the pia mater. The subarachnoid space, located between the arachnoid and the pia mater, contains cerebrospinal fluid.

Pia Mater

The pia mater is the deepest and extremely thin layer that closely follows the brain's surface and tightly covers fissures and sulci. The arachnoid and pia mater together are referred to as the *leptomeninges.*

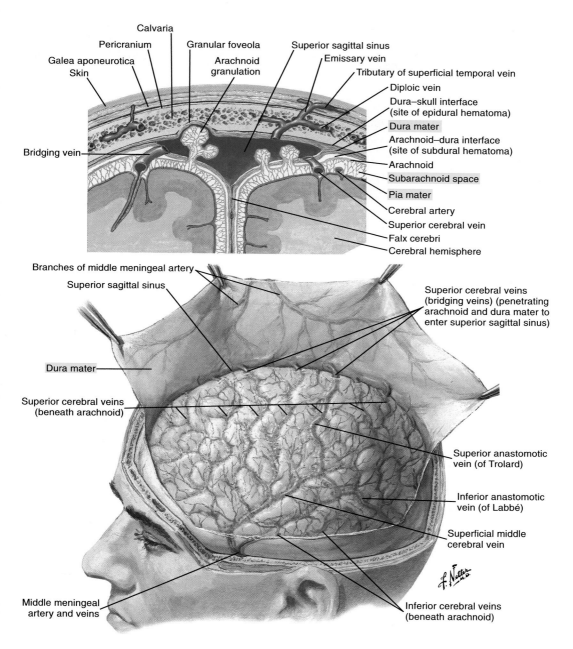

Figure 5-11 The meninges and superficial cerebral veins.

■ CEREBROSPINAL FLUID (Figures 5-12 and 5-13 [p. 226])

The principal source of cerebrospinal fluid is the choroid plexuses in the lateral ventricles, with contributions from other ventricular and extraventricular sites. Cerebrospinal fluid flows from the third and fourth ventricles into the subarachnoid space. It is reabsorbed into the dural venous sinuses and other sites and supports the weight of the brain and provides shock absorption against brain trauma. Cerebrospinal fluid transports nutrients and eliminates waste products.

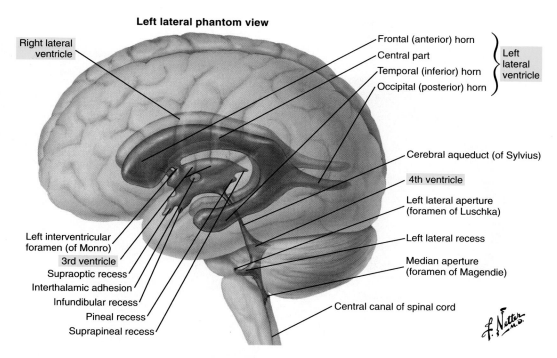

Left lateral phantom view

Right lateral ventricle

Frontal (anterior) horn

Central part

Temporal (inferior) horn

Occipital (posterior) horn

Left lateral ventricle

Cerebral aqueduct (of Sylvius)

4th ventricle

Left lateral aperture (foramen of Luschka)

Left interventricular foramen (of Monro)

3rd ventricle

Supraoptic recess

Interthalamic adhesion

Infundibular recess

Pineal recess

Suprapineal recess

Left lateral recess

Median aperture (foramen of Magendie)

Central canal of spinal cord

Figure 5-12 Ventricles of the brain.

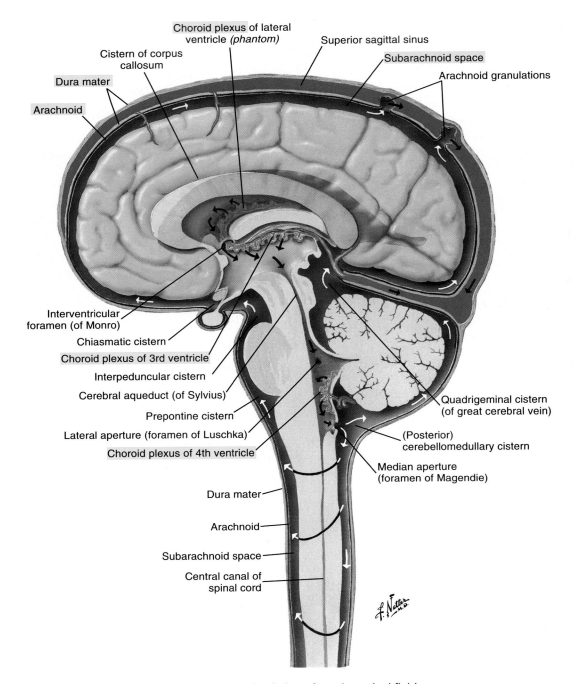

Choroid plexus of lateral
ventricle *(phantom)*

Cistern of corpus
callosum

Dura mater

Arachnoid

Superior sagittal sinus

Subarachnoid space

Arachnoid granulations

Interventricular
foramen (of Monro)

Chiasmatic cistern

Choroid plexus of 3rd ventricle

Interpeduncular cistern

Cerebral aqueduct (of Sylvius)

Prepontine cistern

Lateral aperture (foramen of Luschka)

Choroid plexus of 4th ventricle

Dura mater

Arachnoid

Subarachnoid space

Central canal of
spinal cord

Quadrigeminal cistern
(of great cerebral vein)

(Posterior)
cerebellomedullary cistern

Median aperture
(foramen of Magendie)

Figure 5-13 The circulation of cerebrospinal fluid.

■ CEREBRAL VASCULATURE

Brain tissues have a high metabolic rate, and appropriate blood flow is crucial. The brain consumes approximately 20% of the oxygen supply of the body. Blood supply to the brain comes primarily from the *internal carotid arteries,* which arise from the common carotid, and the *vertebral arteries,* which arise from the subclavian arteries.

The two vertebral arteries, which join to become the basilar artery, supply the brainstem, cerebellum, and occipital lobe. The internal carotid arteries through the anterior, middle, and posterior cerebral arteries supply the cerebral cortex. Cerebral vasculature and the brain regions supplied are shown schematically in Figures 5-14 (p. 228), 5-15 (p. 229), and 5-16 (p. 230).

The *circle of Willis* (Figure 5-17, p. 231) is a key distribution network for blood to the brain. It is formed by the basilar artery, internal carotid arteries, middle cerebral arteries, anterior cerebral arteries, anterior communicating arteries that join the right and left anterior cerebral arteries, and the posterior cerebral arteries that join the internal carotids by the posterior communicating arteries. Thus, through the communicating arteries, this vasculature forms a circle of blood flow to the brain and allows for collateral blood flow in the event of interruptions to cerebral vasculature as the result of disease or damage (e.g., stroke). Most of the venous blood is drained from the venous dural sinuses through the internal jugular veins.

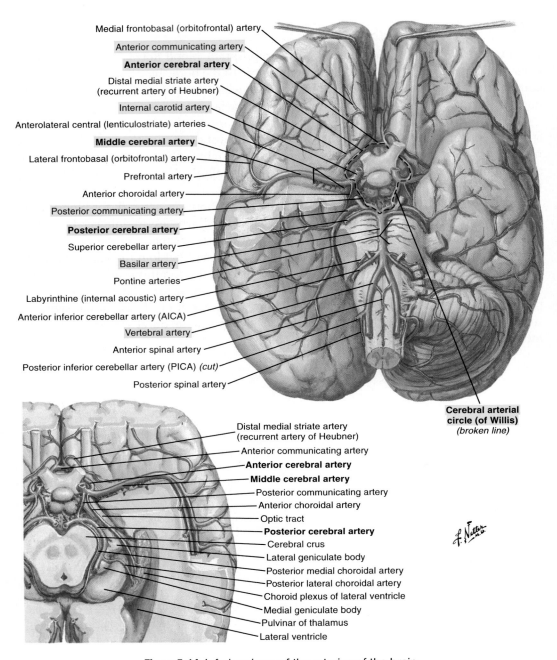

Medial frontobasal (orbitofrontal) artery

Anterior communicating artery

Anterior cerebral artery

Distal medial striate artery
(recurrent artery of Heubner)

Internal carotid artery

Anterolateral central (lenticulostriate) arteries

Middle cerebral artery

Lateral frontobasal (orbitofrontal) artery

Prefrontal artery

Anterior choroidal artery

Posterior communicating artery

Posterior cerebral artery

Superior cerebellar artery

Basilar artery

Pontine arteries

Labyrinthine (internal acoustic) artery

Anterior inferior cerebellar artery (AICA)

Vertebral artery

Anterior spinal artery

Posterior inferior cerebellar artery (PICA) *(cut)*

Posterior spinal artery

**Cerebral arterial
circle (of Willis)**
(broken line)

Distal medial striate artery
(recurrent artery of Heubner)

Anterior communicating artery

Anterior cerebral artery

Middle cerebral artery

Posterior communicating artery

Anterior choroidal artery

Optic tract

Posterior cerebral artery

Cerebral crus

Lateral geniculate body

Posterior medial choroidal artery

Posterior lateral choroidal artery

Choroid plexus of lateral ventricle

Medial geniculate body

Pulvinar of thalamus

Lateral ventricle

Figure 5-14 Inferior views of the arteries of the brain.

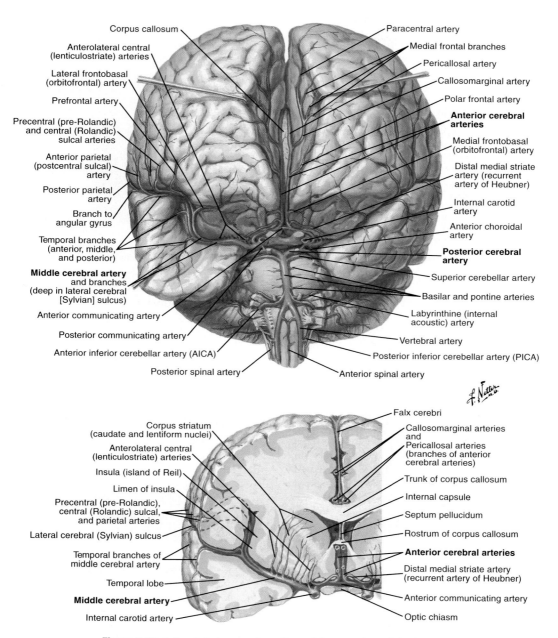

Corpus callosum

Anterolateral central
(lenticulostriate) arteries

Lateral frontobasal
(orbitofrontal) artery

Prefrontal artery

Precentral (pre-Rolandic)
and central (Rolandic)
sulcal arteries

Anterior parietal
(postcentral sulcal)
artery

Posterior parietal
artery

Branch to
angular gyrus

Temporal branches
(anterior, middle,
and posterior)

Middle cerebral artery
and branches
(deep in lateral cerebral
[Sylvian] sulcus)

Anterior communicating artery

Posterior communicating artery

Anterior inferior cerebellar artery (AICA)

Posterior spinal artery

Paracentral artery

Medial frontal branches

Pericallosal artery

Callosomarginal artery

Polar frontal artery

**Anterior cerebral
arteries**

Medial frontobasal
(orbitofrontal) artery

Distal medial striate
artery (recurrent
artery of Heubner)

Internal carotid
artery

Anterior choroidal
artery

**Posterior cerebral
artery**

Superior cerebellar artery

Basilar and pontine arteries

Labyrinthine (internal
acoustic) artery

Vertebral artery

Posterior inferior cerebellar artery (PICA)

Anterior spinal artery

Corpus striatum
(caudate and lentiform nuclei)

Anterolateral central
(lenticulostriate) arteries

Insula (island of Reil)

Limen of insula

Precentral (pre-Rolandic),
central (Rolandic) sulcal,
and parietal arteries

Lateral cerebral (Sylvian) sulcus

Temporal branches of
middle cerebral artery

Temporal lobe

Middle cerebral artery

Internal carotid artery

Falx cerebri

Callosomarginal arteries
and
Pericallosal arteries
(branches of anterior
cerebral arteries)

Trunk of corpus callosum

Internal capsule

Septum pellucidum

Rostrum of corpus callosum

Anterior cerebral arteries

Distal medial striate artery
(recurrent artery of Heubner)

Anterior communicating artery

Optic chiasm

Figure 5-15 A frontal view and section of the arteries of the brain.

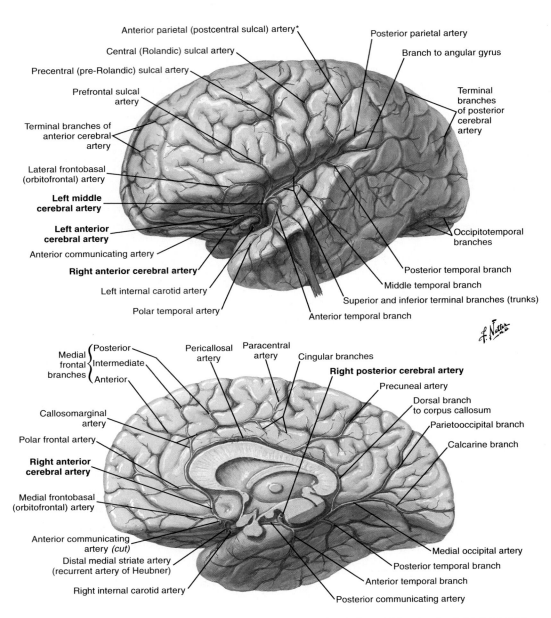

Anterior parietal (postcentral sulcal) artery*

Central (Rolandic) sulcal artery

Precentral (pre-Rolandic) sulcal artery

Prefrontal sulcal artery

Terminal branches of anterior cerebral artery

Lateral frontobasal (orbitofrontal) artery

Left middle cerebral artery

Left anterior cerebral artery

Anterior communicating artery

Right anterior cerebral artery

Left internal carotid artery

Polar temporal artery

Posterior parietal artery

Branch to angular gyrus

Terminal branches of posterior cerebral artery

Occipitotemporal branches

Posterior temporal branch

Middle temporal branch

Superior and inferior terminal branches (trunks)

Anterior temporal branch

Medial frontal branches { Posterior, Intermediate, Anterior }

Pericallosal artery

Paracentral artery

Cingular branches

Right posterior cerebral artery

Precuneal artery

Dorsal branch to corpus callosum

Parietooccipital branch

Calcarine branch

Callosomarginal artery

Polar frontal artery

Right anterior cerebral artery

Medial frontobasal (orbitofrontal) artery

Anterior communicating artery *(cut)*

Distal medial striate artery (recurrent artery of Heubner)

Right internal carotid artery

Medial occipital artery

Posterior temporal branch

Anterior temporal branch

Posterior communicating artery

*Note: Anterior parietal (postcentral sulcal) artery also occurs as separate anterior parietal and postcentral sulcal arteries.

Figure 5-16 Lateral and medial views of the arteries of the brain.

Vessels dissected out: inferior view

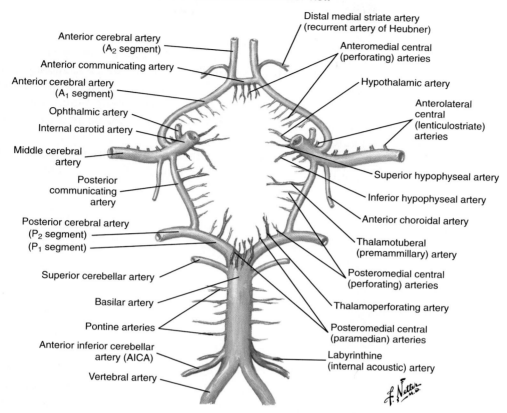

Distal medial striate artery (recurrent artery of Heubner)

Anterior cerebral artery (A_2 segment)

Anterior communicating artery

Anterior cerebral artery (A_1 segment)

Ophthalmic artery

Internal carotid artery

Middle cerebral artery

Posterior communicating artery

Posterior cerebral artery (P_2 segment) (P_1 segment)

Superior cerebellar artery

Basilar artery

Pontine arteries

Anterior inferior cerebellar artery (AICA)

Vertebral artery

Anteromedial central (perforating) arteries

Hypothalamic artery

Anterolateral central (lenticulostriate) arteries

Superior hypophyseal artery

Inferior hypophyseal artery

Anterior choroidal artery

Thalamotuberal (premammillary) artery

Posteromedial central (perforating) arteries

Thalamoperforating artery

Posteromedial central (paramedian) arteries

Labyrinthine (internal acoustic) artery

Figure 5-17 The cerebral arterial circle (of Willis).

■ CRANIAL NERVES (Figure 5-18; see also Figures 5-7 [p. 215], 5-19 [p. 235], 5-20 [p. 239], and 5-26 [p. 251])

Twelve pairs of cranial nerves emerge from the brain, passing through different cranial foramen to innervate structures of the head and neck. Some of these nerves, like the vagus, also innervate structures other than the head and neck such as the thoracic and abdominal cavities. Cranial nerve (and spinal nerve) motoneurons, their axons, and the muscle fibers they innervate form important functional units called *motor units*. Motor units represent the "final common pathway" for the control of movement (as termed by Charles Sherrington, a pioneering neurophysiologist).

Following is a list of all of the cranial nerves. Note that the nerves are numbered using Roman numerals I to XII according to the location of their nuclei, from rostral to caudal.

I   Olfactory
II   Optic
III   Oculomotor
IV   Trochlear
V   Trigeminal
VI   Abducens
VII   Facial
VIII   Vestibulocochlear
IX   Glossopharyngeal
X   Vagus
XI   Accessory
XII   Hypoglossal

The cranial nerve nuclei are located mainly in the brainstem. Mixed nerves (sensory and motor) have more than one nucleus of origin—at least one sensory and one motor. The nuclei of cranial nerves III and IV are located in the midbrain; those of cranial nerves V, VI, VII, and VIII are located in the pons; and those of nerves IX, X, XI, and XII are located in the medulla. Two of the cranial nerve nuclei are not located in the brainstem: the olfactory nerve (I) nucleus, which is located in the telencephalon, and the optic nerve (II) nucleus, which is located in the diencephalon. Of the 12 pairs of nerves, five (III, IV, VI, XI, XII) have a purely motor function; three (I, II, VIII) have a purely sensory function; and four (V, VII, IX, X) have a mixed function, both motor and sensory.

The cell bodies of all the sensory nerves are located inside the brain, in the cranial sensory ganglion, with the exception of the cell bodies of the sensory nerves I and II, which are located inside the organs that they innervate (smell and vision). With the exception of some autonomic motoneurons located outside of ganglions, the cell bodies of motor nerves are located in brainstem nuclei.

Cranial Nerve Nuclei in Brainstem: Schema

Medial dissection

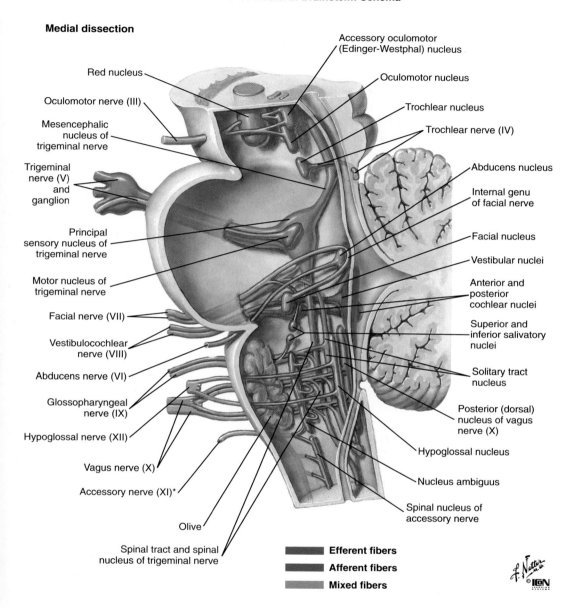

Accessory oculomotor (Edinger-Westphal) nucleus

Red nucleus

Oculomotor nerve (III)

Mesencephalic nucleus of trigeminal nerve

Trigeminal nerve (V) and ganglion

Principal sensory nucleus of trigeminal nerve

Motor nucleus of trigeminal nerve

Facial nerve (VII)

Vestibulocochlear nerve (VIII)

Abducens nerve (VI)

Glossopharyngeal nerve (IX)

Hypoglossal nerve (XII)

Vagus nerve (X)

Accessory nerve (XI)*

Olive

Spinal tract and spinal nucleus of trigeminal nerve

Oculomotor nucleus

Trochlear nucleus

Trochlear nerve (IV)

Abducens nucleus

Internal genu of facial nerve

Facial nucleus

Vestibular nuclei

Anterior and posterior cochlear nuclei

Superior and inferior salivatory nuclei

Solitary tract nucleus

Posterior (dorsal) nucleus of vagus nerve (X)

Hypoglossal nucleus

Nucleus ambiguus

Spinal nucleus of accessory nerve

- Efferent fibers
- Afferent fibers
- Mixed fibers

*Recent evidence suggests that the accessory nerve lacks a cranial root and has no connection to the vagus nerve. Verification of this finding awaits further investigation.

Figure 5-18 A lateral view of the cranial nerve nuclei fiber pathways in the brainstem.

Types of Cranial Nerve Fibers (Figure 5-19)

Cranial nerves can carry up to six functionally distinct types of fibers: three types of sensory fibers and three types of motor fibers. The terms *afferent* for sensory and *efferent* for motor are often used.

Sensory
- General sensory fibers carry touch, pain, temperature, and proprioception.
- Special sensory fibers carry hearing, balance, vision, taste, and smell; they are sometimes divided into special somatic (hearing, vision, and equilibrium) and special visceral (smell and taste).
- Visceral sensory fibers carry sensory information (except pain) from the viscera.

Motor
- Somatic motor fibers innervate somatic skeletal muscles.
- Branchial motor fibers innervate skeletal muscles that develop from the branchial arches (branchiomeric).
- Visceral motor (parasympathetic efferent) fibers innervate smooth muscle and glands.

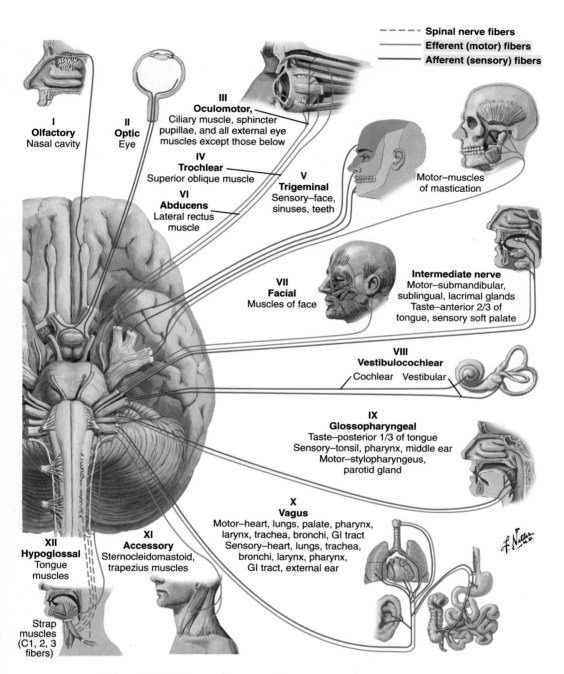

Figure 5-19 Motor and sensory distribution of the cranial nerves.

I Olfactory (Sensory)

The olfactory nerve originates from the olfactory receptors, which are located in the region of the nasal mucosa. The nerve fibers project up through the cribriform plate of the ethmoid bone and synapse on the olfactory bulb. Olfactory fibers travel caudally through the olfactory tract, which runs underneath the frontal lobe; pass into the cerebral hemispheres; and terminate in the primary olfactory area, in the medial temporal lobe.

The brain exit point of cranial nerve I is the telencephalon, and the cranial exit point is the cribriform plate of the ethmoid bone. Function is special sensory: olfaction.

II Optic (Sensory)

The optic nerve originates from the retina. Its fibers course within the optic canal, which is formed by the posterior portion of the sphenoid bone, and converge to form the optic chiasm. The fibers then diverge into the optic tracts, which course toward the thalamus, where the fibers synapse. The nerve fibers leave the thalamus to travel to the primary visual area in the occipital cortex.

The brain exit point of cranial nerve II is the diencephalon, and the cranial exit point is the optic foramen. Function is special sensory: vision.

III Oculomotor (Motor)

The oculomotor nerve originates from the anterior part of the mesencephalon and travels within the orbit to reach the eye. The brain exit point of cranial nerve III is the mesencephalon, and the cranial exit point is the supraorbital fissure of the sphenoid bone.

Function is motor, as follows:

- Somatic motor: to the six extraocular eye muscles and the levator muscle of upper eyelid.
- Visceral motor: to the constrictor pupillae and ciliary muscles that are involved in the pupillary light and accommodation reflexes.

IV Trochlear (Motor)

The smallest cranial nerve originates from the posterior area of the mesencephalon at the level of the inferior colliculus. Its fibers circle around the brainstem and course forward toward the eye in the subarachnoid space. The brain exit point of cranial nerve IV is the mesencephalon, and the cranial exit point is the superior orbital fissure. The function of this nerve is somatic motor to the superior oblique muscle in the orbit.

V Trigeminal (Motor and Sensory) (Figure 5-20)

The trigeminal nerves are the largest cranial nerves and are composed of three main divisions: ophthalmic, maxillary, and mandibular. The roots converge at the level of the petrous portion of the temporal bone to form the trigeminal ganglion. The trigeminal nerve courses from the pons to the face. The brain exit point is the metencephalon (pons).

Ophthalmic Nerve, or Branch (V₁) (Sensory)

The cranial exit point of the ophthalmic nerve is the supraorbital fissure of the sphenoid bone.

   Function is as follows:

- General sensory: from the sinuses, skin of the forehead, upper eyelid, and nose; mucous membranes of nasal cavity; short and long ciliary nerves of the eye (iris and cornea).
- Visceral sensory: from the lacrimal gland.

Maxillary Nerve, or Branch (V₂) (Sensory)

The cranial exit point of the maxillary nerve is the foramen rotundum of the sphenoid bone. Function is general sensory: from the dura mater, skin of the side of the forehead, cheeks, lower eyelid, upper lip, upper teeth, maxilla, palate, nasal septum and posterior portion of nasal cavity, and gums and mucous membranes of the oral cavity.

Mandibular Nerve, or Branch (V₃) (Sensory and Motor)

The cranial exit point of the mandibular nerve is the foramen ovale of the sphenoid bone.

   Function is as follows:

- General sensory: from the anterior two-thirds of the tongue, mucous membranes of the mouth, the mandible, the lower teeth, lower lip, the chin, part of the external ear and cheek, and meninges of anterior and middle cranial fossae.
- Branchial motor: to the muscles of mastication, the tensor tympani muscle, and the tensor veli palatini.

Mesencephalic Trigeminal Nucleus (MesV)

Primary sensory neurons carry proprioceptive sensory information from the masticatory muscles and project primarily to the trigeminal motor nucleus for reflex control of masticatory movements.

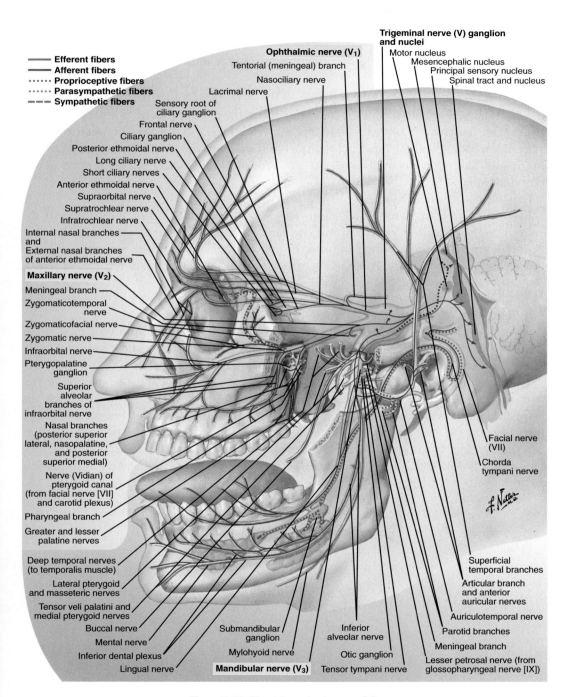

Trigeminal nerve (V) ganglion and nuclei
- Motor nucleus
- Mesencephalic nucleus
- Principal sensory nucleus
- Spinal tract and nucleus

Ophthalmic nerve (V₁)
- Tentorial (meningeal) branch
- Nasociliary nerve
- Lacrimal nerve

—— Efferent fibers
—— Afferent fibers
······ Proprioceptive fibers
······ Parasympathetic fibers
− − − Sympathetic fibers

Sensory root of ciliary ganglion
Frontal nerve
Ciliary ganglion
Posterior ethmoidal nerve
Long ciliary nerve
Short ciliary nerves
Anterior ethmoidal nerve
Supraorbital nerve
Supratrochlear nerve
Infratrochlear nerve
Internal nasal branches and
External nasal branches of anterior ethmoidal nerve

Maxillary nerve (V₂)

Meningeal branch
Zygomaticotemporal nerve
Zygomaticofacial nerve
Zygomatic nerve
Infraorbital nerve
Pterygopalatine ganglion
Superior alveolar branches of infraorbital nerve
Nasal branches (posterior superior lateral, nasopalatine, and posterior superior medial)
Nerve (Vidian) of pterygoid canal (from facial nerve [VII] and carotid plexus)
Pharyngeal branch
Greater and lesser palatine nerves

Deep temporal nerves (to temporalis muscle)
Lateral pterygoid and masseteric nerves
Tensor veli palatini and medial pterygoid nerves
Buccal nerve
Mental nerve
Inferior dental plexus
Lingual nerve

Submandibular ganglion
Mylohyoid nerve
Mandibular nerve (V₃)

Inferior alveolar nerve
Otic ganglion
Tensor tympani nerve

Facial nerve (VII)
Chorda tympani nerve

Superficial temporal branches
Articular branch and anterior auricular nerves
Auriculotemporal nerve
Parotid branches
Meningeal branch
Lesser petrosal nerve (from glossopharyngeal nerve [IX])

Figure 5-20 The trigeminal nerve (V).

VI Abducens (Motor)

The abducens nerve originates from the inferior part of the pons and penetrates into the orbit to reach the eye. The brain exit point is the junction between the metencephalon and the myelencephalon, and the cranial exit point is the supraorbital fissure of the sphenoid bone.

Function is somatic motor: to the lateral rectus muscle of the ipsilateral orbit.

VII Facial (Motor and Sensory) (Figure 5-21)

The facial nerve originates from the pons and enters the temporal bone to emerge from the cranium as five distinct branches. The brain exit point is the junction between the metencephalon (pons) and the myelencephalon. For the cranial exit point, the nerve runs in the internal auditory meatus and leaves the skull through the stylomastoid foramen of the temporal bone.

Function is mixed, as follows:
- General sensory: from the skin behind the external ear and skin of the concha of the auricle, external auditory meatus, and tympanic membrane (external surface).
- Special sensory: taste information from the anterior two-thirds of the tongue.
- Branchial motor: to muscles of facial expression (but not the primary muscles of mastication), as well as the stapedius muscle.
- Visceral motor: to the mucous membranes of hard and soft palate and nose, as well as lacrimal, submandibular, and sublingual glands.

Several terminal branches of the facial nerves join to form the parotid plexus, which is located in the parotid salivary gland. The nerve passes into the gland and divides into several branches: temporal, zygomatic, buccal, mandibular, and cervical.

The motor component of the facial nerve contains two segments: one that originates from the superior portion of the facial nerve nuclei and innervates the superior portion of the face and one that originates from the inferior portion of the facial nerve nuclei and innervates the inferior portion of the face. The superior portions of the nerve that innervate the superior portions of the face receive input from both hemispheres. In contrast, the inferior portions that innervate the lower portion of the face receive only contralateral cortical input.

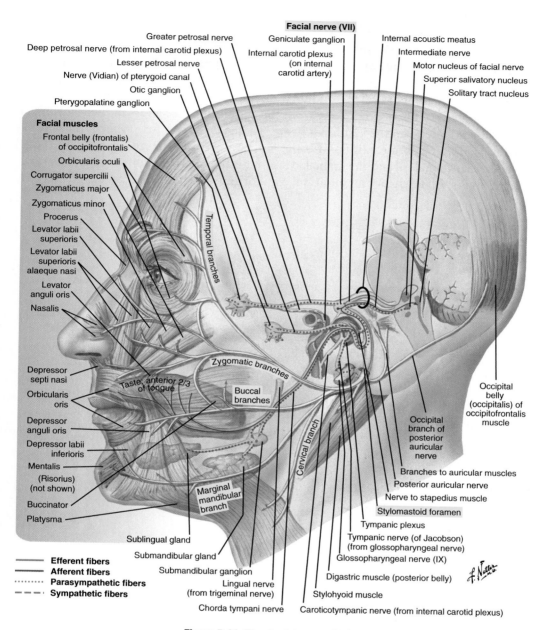

Figure 5-21 The facial nerve (VII).

VIII Vestibulocochlear (Sensory) (Figure 5-22)

The vestibulocochlear nerve originates from the internal ear, is located in the temporal bone, runs through the internal auditory meatus, and terminates in the brainstem at the level of the junction between the metencephalon (pons) and the myelencephalon. The nerve fibers originating from the auditory receptors in the cochlea form the cochlear nerve, and the nerve fibers originating from the equilibrium receptors in the semicircular canals and vestibule form the vestibular nerve. These two nerves fuse to form the vestibulocochlear nerve. The brain exit point is the junction between the metencephalon (pons) and the myelencephalon, and the cranial exit point is the internal auditory meatus.

Function is special sensory for audition, equilibrium, and body orientation.

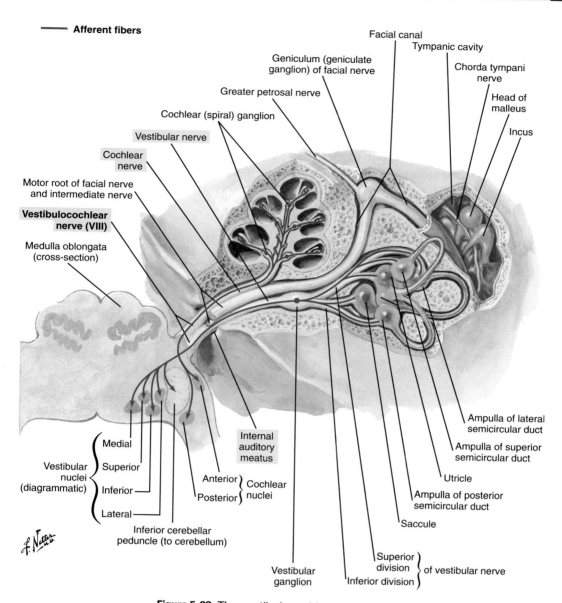

Afferent fibers

Facial canal
Tympanic cavity
Geniculum (geniculate ganglion) of facial nerve
Chorda tympani nerve
Greater petrosal nerve
Head of malleus
Cochlear (spiral) ganglion
Incus
Vestibular nerve
Cochlear nerve
Motor root of facial nerve and intermediate nerve
Vestibulocochlear nerve (VIII)
Medulla oblongata (cross-section)

Ampulla of lateral semicircular duct
Ampulla of superior semicircular duct
Medial
Vestibular nuclei (diagrammatic)
Superior
Inferior
Lateral
Internal auditory meatus
Anterior
Posterior
Cochlear nuclei
Utricle
Ampulla of posterior semicircular duct
Saccule
Inferior cerebellar peduncle (to cerebellum)
Vestibular ganglion
Superior division
Inferior division
of vestibular nerve

Figure 5-22 The vestibulocochlear nerve (VIII).

IX Glossopharyngeal (Motor and Sensory) (Figure 5-23)

The glossopharyngeal nerve originates from the myelencephalon and courses from the cranium to the pharynx. The brain exit point of cranial nerve IX is the myelencephalon, and the cranial exit point is the jugular foramen, between the temporal bone and the occipital bone.

Function is mixed, as follows:

- Branchial motor: to the stylopharyngeus muscle.
- Visceral motor: to the parotid gland.
- General sensory: from the posterior one-third of the tongue, the tonsils, the pharynx, tympanic membrane (internal surface), the tympanic cavity, eustachian tube, and the skin of the external ear.
- Visceral sensory: from the carotid body and sinus.
- Special sensory: taste from the posterior one-third of the tongue.

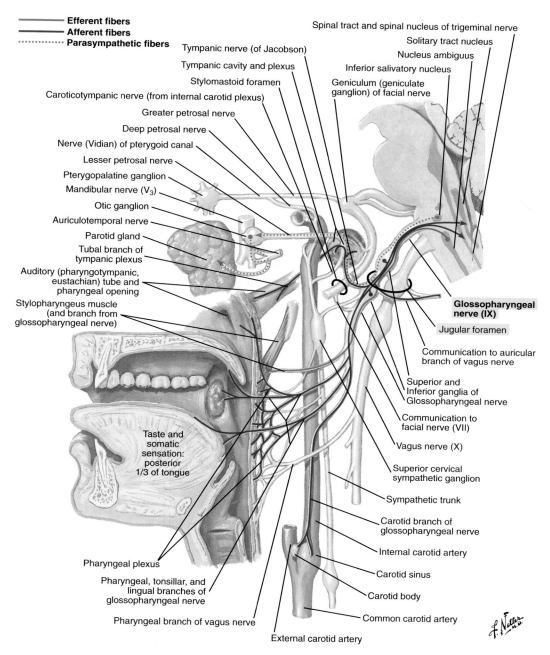

Efferent fibers
Afferent fibers
Parasympathetic fibers

Tympanic nerve (of Jacobson)
Tympanic cavity and plexus
Stylomastoid foramen
Caroticotympanic nerve (from internal carotid plexus)
Greater petrosal nerve
Deep petrosal nerve
Nerve (Vidian) of pterygoid canal
Lesser petrosal nerve
Pterygopalatine ganglion
Mandibular nerve (V₃)
Otic ganglion
Auriculotemporal nerve
Parotid gland
Tubal branch of tympanic plexus
Auditory (pharyngotympanic, eustachian) tube and pharyngeal opening
Stylopharyngeus muscle (and branch from glossopharyngeal nerve)

Spinal tract and spinal nucleus of trigeminal nerve
Solitary tract nucleus
Nucleus ambiguus
Inferior salivatory nucleus
Geniculum (geniculate ganglion) of facial nerve

Glossopharyngeal nerve (IX)
Jugular foramen
Communication to auricular branch of vagus nerve
Superior and Inferior ganglia of Glossopharyngeal nerve
Communication to facial nerve (VII)
Vagus nerve (X)
Superior cervical sympathetic ganglion
Sympathetic trunk
Carotid branch of glossopharyngeal nerve
Internal carotid artery
Carotid sinus
Carotid body
Common carotid artery

Taste and somatic sensation: posterior 1/3 of tongue

Pharyngeal plexus
Pharyngeal, tonsillar, and lingual branches of glossopharyngeal nerve
Pharyngeal branch of vagus nerve
External carotid artery

Figure 5-23 The glossopharyngeal nerve (IX).

X Vagus, or Pneumogastric, Nerve (Motor and Sensory) (Figure 5-24)

The vagus nerve originates from the medulla; travels down to the jugular foramen; and continues its course down to the neck, thorax, and abdomen. The brain exit point is the myelencephalon, and the cranial exit point is the jugular foramen, between the temporal bone and the occipital bone.

Function is mixed, as follows:

- Branchial motor: to muscles of the pharynx (except the stylopharyngeus, which is innervated by the glossopharyngeal nerve), muscles of the larynx, and muscles of the soft palate (except the tensor veli palatini, which is innervated by the trigeminal nerve).
- Visceral motor: to smooth muscle and glands of the pharynx, larynx, and viscera of the thorax and abdomen, including smooth muscle of the esophagus and cardiac muscle.
- General sensory: from portions of the skin of the external ear and auditory canal, part of the external surface of the tympanic membrane, the pharynx and larynx, and meninges of posterior cranial fossa.
- Visceral sensory: from the larynx (above and below the vocal folds), esophagus, trachea, heart, and thoracic and abdominal viscera (including the lungs and gastrointestinal tract).

Vagus Nerve (X): Schema

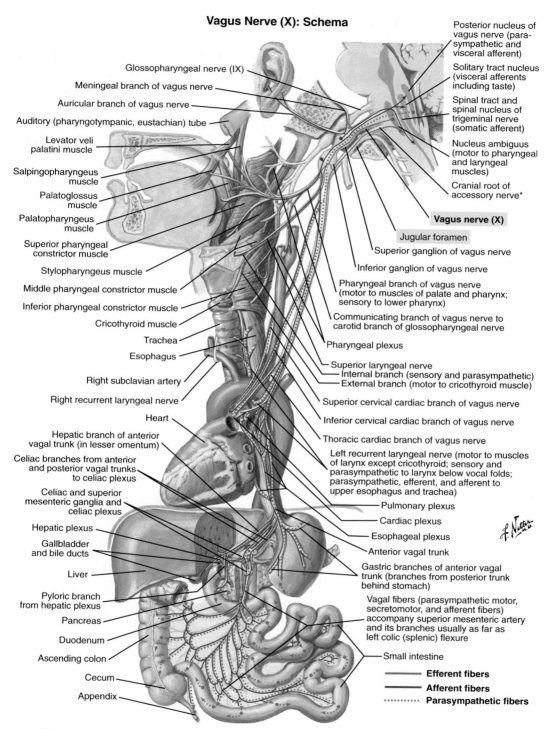

Glossopharyngeal nerve (IX)

Meningeal branch of vagus nerve

Auricular branch of vagus nerve

Auditory (pharyngotympanic, eustachian) tube

Levator veli palatini muscle

Salpingopharyngeus muscle

Palatoglossus muscle

Palatopharyngeus muscle

Superior pharyngeal constrictor muscle

Stylopharyngeus muscle

Middle pharyngeal constrictor muscle

Inferior pharyngeal constrictor muscle

Cricothyroid muscle

Trachea

Esophagus

Right subclavian artery

Right recurrent laryngeal nerve

Heart

Hepatic branch of anterior vagal trunk (in lesser omentum)

Celiac branches from anterior and posterior vagal trunks to celiac plexus

Celiac and superior mesenteric ganglia and celiac plexus

Hepatic plexus

Gallbladder and bile ducts

Liver

Pyloric branch from hepatic plexus

Pancreas

Duodenum

Ascending colon

Cecum

Appendix

Posterior nucleus of vagus nerve (parasympathetic and visceral afferent)

Solitary tract nucleus (visceral afferents including taste)

Spinal tract and spinal nucleus of trigeminal nerve (somatic afferent)

Nucleus ambiguus (motor to pharyngeal and laryngeal muscles)

Cranial root of accessory nerve*

Vagus nerve (X)

Jugular foramen

Superior ganglion of vagus nerve

Inferior ganglion of vagus nerve

Pharyngeal branch of vagus nerve (motor to muscles of palate and pharynx; sensory to lower pharynx)

Communicating branch of vagus nerve to carotid branch of glossopharyngeal nerve

Pharyngeal plexus

Superior laryngeal nerve
Internal branch (sensory and parasympathetic)
External branch (motor to cricothyroid muscle)

Superior cervical cardiac branch of vagus nerve

Inferior cervical cardiac branch of vagus nerve

Thoracic cardiac branch of vagus nerve

Left recurrent laryngeal nerve (motor to muscles of larynx except cricothyroid; sensory and parasympathetic to larynx below vocal folds; parasympathetic, efferent, and afferent to upper esophagus and trachea)

Pulmonary plexus

Cardiac plexus

Esophageal plexus

Anterior vagal trunk

Gastric branches of anterior vagal trunk (branches from posterior trunk behind stomach)

Vagal fibers (parasympathetic motor, secretomotor, and afferent fibers) accompany superior mesenteric artery and its branches usually as far as left colic (splenic) flexure

Small intestine

———— **Efferent fibers**

———— **Afferent fibers**

·············· **Parasympathetic fibers**

*Recent evidence suggests that the accessory nerve lacks a cranial root and has no connection to the vagus nerve. Verification of this finding awaits further investigation.

Figure 5-24 The vagus nerve (X).

XI Accessory (Motor) (Figure 5-25)

The accessory nerve originates from the union of a cranial root and a spinal root. The accessory nerve exits the skull through the jugular foramen, between the temporal bone and the occipital bone. The cranial fibers quickly branch off to join the vagus nerve; the spinal fibers travel backward and downward to join the large skeletal muscles of the neck. The brain exit point is the myelencephalon, and the cranial exit point is the jugular foramen, between the temporal bone and the occipital bone.

Function is branchial motor: the spinal branch innervates the trapezius and sternocleidomastoid muscles. The cranial branch that joins the vagus nerve innervates the larynx, the pharynx, and the soft palate (see the section on the Vagus Nerve, p. 246).

Accessory Nerve (XI): Schema

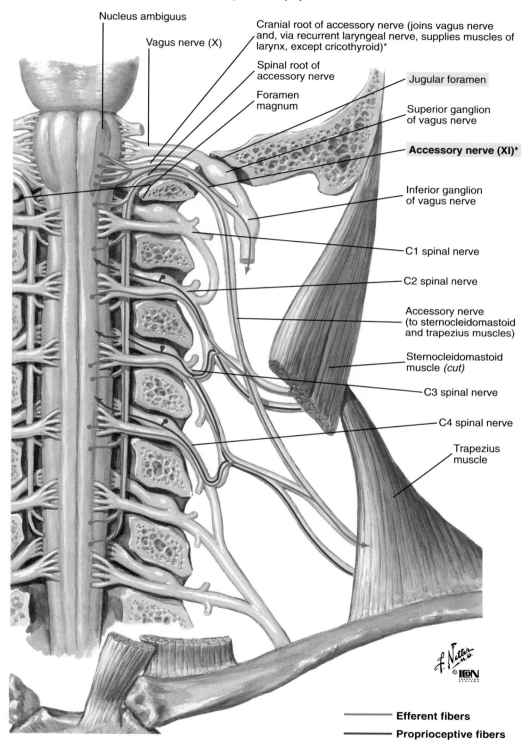

Nucleus ambiguus

Vagus nerve (X)

Cranial root of accessory nerve (joins vagus nerve and, via recurrent laryngeal nerve, supplies muscles of larynx, except cricothyroid)*

Spinal root of accessory nerve

Foramen magnum

Jugular foramen

Superior ganglion of vagus nerve

Accessory nerve (XI)*

Inferior ganglion of vagus nerve

C1 spinal nerve

C2 spinal nerve

Accessory nerve (to sternocleidomastoid and trapezius muscles)

Sternocleidomastoid muscle *(cut)*

C3 spinal nerve

C4 spinal nerve

Trapezius muscle

——— Efferent fibers

——— Proprioceptive fibers

*Recent evidence suggests that the accessory nerve lacks a cranial root and has no connection to the vagus nerve. Verification of this finding awaits further investigation.

Figure 5-25 The accessory nerve (XI).

XII Hypoglossal (Motor) (Figure 5-26)

The hypoglossal nerve originates from the medulla and innervates the muscles of the tongue. The brain exit point of cranial nerve XII is the myelencephalon, and the cranial exit point is the hypoglossal canal in the occipital bone.

Function is branchial motor: to all intrinsic muscles of the tongue and three of the four extrinsic muscles of the tongue—genioglossus, styloglossus, and hyoglossus. The fourth muscle, the palatoglossus, is supplied by the vagus nerve. The hypoglossal nerve also supplies the sternothyroid, sternohyoid, thyrohyoid, genioglossus, geniohyoid, mylohyoid, and anterior belly of the omohyoid.

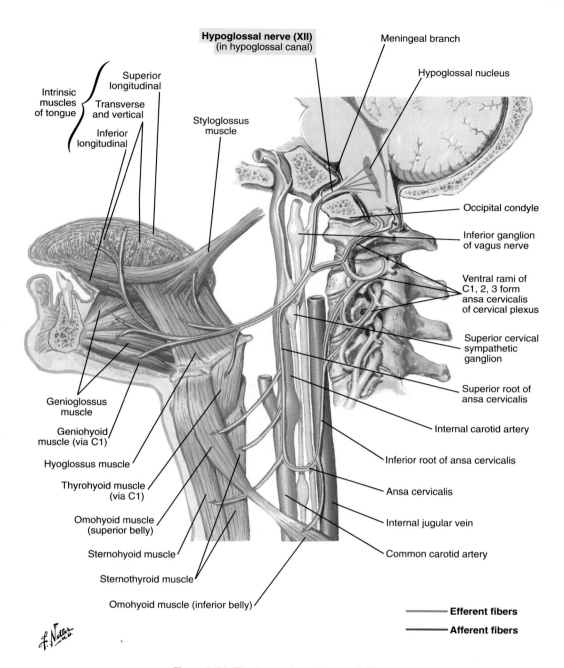

Figure 5-26 The hypoglossal nerve (XII).

Summary of Cranial Nerves Significant to Speech, Mastication/Swallowing, and Hearing

Cranial Nerve	Structure Supplied
V Trigeminal (sensory/motor) (see Figure 5-20, p. 239) Three branches: 1. Ophthalmic 2. Maxillary 3. Mandibular	*Sensory:* from the face, mouth, palate, teeth, nasal cavity, and anterior two-thirds of the tongue *Motor:* to the muscles of mastication (except for the posterior belly of the digastric and geniohyoid), muscles of the floor of the mouth, and tensor veli palatini and tensor tympani
VII Facial (sensory/motor)(see Figure 5-21, p. 241)	*Motor:* to muscles of facial expression and nasal muscles, posterior belly of the digastric, stylohyoid, and stapedius muscle; responsible for facial muscle tone *Secretory:* for the lacrimal, submandibular, and sublingual glands and mucous membranes for palate and nose *Taste:* from anterior two-thirds of the tongue
VIII Vestibulocochlear (sensory/motor) (see Figure 5-22, p. 243)	*Sensory:* from auditory (cochlear branch) and equilibrium (vestibular branch)
IX Glossopharyngeal (sensory/motor) (see Figure 5-23, p. 245)	*Sensory:* from the posterior one-third of the tongue, pharynx, tonsils, internal surface of tympanic membrane, tympanic cavity, eustachian tube *Motor:* to the stylopharyngeus muscle *Secretory:* for the parotid gland *Taste:* from the posterior one-third of the tongue
X Vagus (sensory/motor) (see Figure 5-24, p. 247)	*Sensory:* from larynx and pharynx, thorax, abdomen, external surface of tympanic membrane, part of external ear and auditory canal *Motor:* to intrinsic laryngeal (except stylopharyngeus), soft palate (except for the tensor veli palatini), and esophageal muscles *Taste:* from the epiglottic region and the root of the tongue
XI Accessory (motor) (see Figure 5-25, p. 249)	*Motor:* to trapezius and sternocleidomastoid
XII Hypoglossal (motor) (see Figure 5-26, p. 251)	*Motor:* to all intrinsic and most extrinsic muscles of the tongue (except the palatoglossus), some suprahyoid, including the geniohyoid muscle and infrahyoid muscles (sternohyoid, omohyoid, sternothyroid, thyrohyoid)

INDEX

Page numbers followed by *f,* indicate figures; *t,* tables; *b,* boxes.